Breaking Your Fat Girl Habits

Breaking Your Fat Girl Habits

Weight loss mistakes even healthy chicks make!

Danielle Pashko

Copyright © 2015 Danielle Pashko
All rights reserved.

ISBN: 1514759543
ISBN 13: 9781514759547
Library of Congress Control Number: 2015910453
CreateSpace Independent Publishing Platform
North Charleston, South Carolina

*I dedicate this book to ladies everywhere.
My wish is to empower you with the knowledge
to achieve the body you've always wanted.*

*I would like to also acknowledge
the advice and encouragement of the following people:*

My mentor, colleague, and dear friend Oz Garcia and the rest of our office team - Albert, Freddy, Tara, Claudia, Margaret and Samir for all of their support; all of my awesome experts who contributed - Mike Mutzel (author of Belly Fat Effect*), Brett Hoebel (one of the most amazing fitness trainers in the world), Dr. Lionel Bissoon (a leading physician on Anti-Aging medicine); and Christina Hamlett (my editor, who is also a great friend and like a big sister).*

TABLE OF CONTENTS

Foreword · ix
Introduction · xi
Chapter 1: Identifying Your Fat Girl Habits · · · · · · · · · · 1
Chapter 2: Change Your Beliefs, Change Your Body · · · · · · 6
Chapter 3: Stop Stressing · 11
Chapter 4: What's in a Portion? · · · · · · · · · · · · · · · · 16
Chapter 5: Don't Waste a Workout · · · · · · · · · · · · · · 22
Chapter 6: You Are Not a Sumo Wrestler · · · · · · · · · · · 29
Chapter 7: Protein is a Girl's Best Friend · · · · · · · · · · · 35
Chapter 8: Vegetarian Doesn't = Skinny · · · · · · · · · · · 41
Chapter 9: Gluten-Free Mistakes You Don't Want to Make · · · · · · 48
Chapter 10: The Dark Side of Juicing · · · · · · · · · · · · · 53
Chapter 11: Snacks That Can Sabotage or Keep You Skinny · · · · · · 57
Chapter 12: What's Lurking in Your Sauces,
    Dressings and Condiments? · · · · · · · · · · · · · · · 62
Chapter 13: Got Cellulite? · · · · · · · · · · · · · · · · · · · 67
Chapter 14: Weight Loss Slip Ups: Tips From a Hollywood Trainer · · 72
Chapter 15: Oh the Joy of Hormones · · · · · · · · · · · · · 77
Chapter 16: Uncovering Food Sensitivities · · · · · · · · · · 83
Chapter 17: Big Belly – Bad Bacteria · · · · · · · · · · · · · 91
Chapter 18: The Plight of the Orthorexic · · · · · · · · · · · 96
Chapter 19: How to Party Without Paying For It · · · · · · · 102
Chapter 20: The Right Track to Success · · · · · · · · · · · 107

FOREWORD

How many years have you spent killing yourself at the gym and you still haven't reached your goal of a well toned body? How many diet books are currently on your bookshelves – (you should hold your Ph.D in nutrition at this point) - but still can't find a solution to losing weight?

You're not alone in the quest for slimness. On average, dieters make four to five attempts per year – usually in the context of a New Year's resolution, an upcoming school reunion or re-entering the dating pool after divorce. If their expectations aren't realistic, however (*"I'm going to lose 30 pounds in the next two weeks!"*), it's all too easy to get depressed and quit, reverting to the very habits that brought on the problem to begin with.

When it comes to first impressions, the world out there can be pretty harsh about exterior looks. The U.S. may not be the most obsessed about weight but it does have the highest per capita population that weighs more than is healthy or attractive. According to recent statistics by the National Weight Control Registry, over 108 million Americans are on diets, 85 percent of whom are females. Combine this with diet drugs, metabolism-revving protein shakes, celebrity endorsements and weight-loss surgeries such as bariatric and liposuction and you're looking at a $20 billion industry.

So with all these resources at your disposal – and assuming they're within your budget - why are you still dismayed when you see yourself in the mirror? The answer may be that embracing a new weight-loss regimen isn't as easy as reading a recipe in a cookbook or following someone's health blog; you must also take a hard look at the rituals of a lifetime that have led you to believe (1) drinks with friends after work don't count as actual calories, (2) strenuous workouts exclude you from watching your portions (3) anything purchased from the health food store (Organic, Gluten-Free, Vegan, Raw, Non-GMO) can be eaten without discretion.

Fresh on the heels of her first book, *Smile at Your Challenges*, fitness and nutrition expert Danielle Pashko shares insights and professional advice on how to lose self-defeating behaviors…and lose inches and pounds in the process! While one might initially think that someone as tall and sleek as Danielle has never worried about excess weight a single day in her life, she candidly shares that women who are model-thin obsess just as much about body image as those who are on the chunky side. The correlations to self-confidence and self-esteem are further tied to the universal desire to attract a soul mate that finds one's looks appealing.

The biggest takeaway in Danielle's new book, however, is the emphasis on living a healthy lifestyle. You can whittle yourself down to a size 0 but if you're constantly plagued by migraines, irritable bowel syndrome, fatigue, depression and erratic mood swings, is there a possibility that purposefully adjusting your attitude toward food and exercise could make a world of difference? Within these pages, you'll learn how to effect positive change, both internal and external.

For any weight-loss objectives to be successfully met, Danielle believes that you have to hold yourself personally accountable — especially if you're not enrolled in a boot camp with a vigilant drill sergeant or tucked into a lock-down spa retreat where you don't have access to a refrigerator for those midnight snack attacks. Although cheating on a diet or skipping a gym workout is something that anyone can make excuses for, the bigger issue is how much you're cheating yourself out of a more energized body, a cleaner system and an optimistic mindset that anything is possible if you have the discipline to stick with it!

~ **Oz Garcia**, **author of** *Redesigning 50, The Balance, Look and Feel Fabulous Forever, and The Food Cure for Kids*

INTRODUCTION

If my title offends you, that wasn't my intention. I'm just going to be honest at the expense of sounding shallow. Basically every girl I've ever met has aspired to be thin and beautiful. While inner beauty is certainly more important than outer beauty, we are taught from a young age that thin is in. All the female leads in movies, television and even cartoons are always slim and pretty. The matriarchs and fair maidens of stories that have been passed down throughout the generations were always stunning whether they were tall and lean or blessed with big breasts and curvy figures. Magazines and billboards routinely bombard us with images of sleek and slender beauties. And let's not forget that the popular girls at school or the cheerleaders who the guys fall over never fail to have the rocking bodies. So if you were one of those girls that were overweight, life may have been harder for you. As an attempt to fix those issues or be accepted, you may have been pulled into disordered eating, bad habits or poor self-image that doesn't always disappear once you've reached adulthood. The competitiveness just gets more aggressive with age because women will always be catty and men can't help but be visual.

Globally, there are currently more than a billion overweight adults, a scary number that continues to climb. In the U.S. alone, the weight loss market is a $60 billion industry that emphasizes dieting, drugs, supplements, pre-packaged foods and shakes, cosmetic treatments and weight-loss surgery if all else fails. The number of gyms, yoga, Pilates and Spin® centers are gaining cult followings, as are purchases of home exercise equipment and hard core work out videos like Insanity® and P90X® for those who prefer the convenience or are self-conscious about sweating off calories in public. Further, it's hard to channel-surf or read a gossip column and not see before-and-after pictures of individuals (including celebrities) that appear to have been lucky or bombing after attempting to lose weight. While many of the old school programs such as Weight Watchers,™ Jenny Craig™ and Nutri-Systems™ were all the rage, now it's shifted to the modern day juice cleanses, gluten-free, Paleo, or plant-based diets. Let's also not forget about wearable technology and customized apps. The reality, however, is that anything touted as a quick-fix solution to vanquishing fat may work for the short-term but it's the ingrained habits of a lifetime that can just as quickly undo whatever progress was made.

While we know that carrying extra pounds around can potentially invite serious health risks, the paradox is that food as a reward mechanism was likely used by our parents and teachers from the time we were children. Accordingly, we start at a young age to equate fast food, snacks, candy, and unhealthy treats with being special. You have a birthday party, you get a cupcake. You score an A on a test, you get jelly beans. You win the spelling bee and the family takes you out for pizza to celebrate. On the flipside, food can be used to express love when you are feeling upset. You get a booboo and your parents take you for a milkshake. Your sixth grade crush asks someone else to the school dance and you cry to your mother over a tub of ice cream. Food is always to "go to" for emotional support.

I was never what you would call "fat," but I definitely let the idea of being thin consume me starting as a little girl. I began watching my weight around the age of 11 years old because I wanted to be skinny like the other girls in school. I was not yet athletic like I am now and my stepfather would often tease me about being a little chubby or clumsy. His son was the star jock that he clearly favored. We had a turbulent relationship, yet the only way we bonded was over food. He was Italian and a great chef. Cooking for me was the only way I saw his efforts towards having a relationship. He would prepare bowls of pasta or lasagna, keep cakes around the house and always convince me to have seconds. I would go through this cycle of pleasure followed by shame. Eating was much more fun to me that going outside to play with friends.

I still didn't let being a little overweight bother me until another year or so when I started worrying about what the boys thought. I was very tall and already towering over the ones in my grade. I started to feel like a linebacker next to these scrawny little guys! This was when my experimentation with dieting started.

I had no clue what I was doing. My best attempt was just to eat much less and to the point that I was always hungry. I also began excessively exercising from joining the basketball and track teams with their grueling practices. It wasn't easy, though. I felt restricted and would constantly obsess about what went into my mouth even when I was doing activities totally unrelated to food. My kitchen was stocked with rice cakes, diet soda, fat-free popcorn, sugar-free yogurt, fat-free cottage cheese, and cans of tuna. My girlfriends and I used to make runs to 7-Eleven after school to fill up on coffee since it had no calories. We would then add all of those sugar-free creamers with non-fat whipped cream and Sweet'n Low.™ We also experimented with diet pills and laxatives which could potentially make or break my mood after looking at the scale every morning. I definitely had my moments where I would binge on pizza or M&M's™ but then would anxiously weigh myself the next day hoping not to feel terrible. By my senior year I even took up smoking cigarettes.

This wasn't to be cool or fit in, however; I actually smoked in secret as a way to cut my appetite.

My unhealthy methods for keeping the weight off seemed to work through high school but they didn't come without consequences. I completely screwed up my menstrual cycle from swearing off fat. I would get my period twice a year if I was lucky. My metabolism started to shut down from not eating regularly and it seemed that if I ate more than a bird I would gain weight.

Following graduation I wasn't playing sports the way I used to. That meant I now had to find another method of exercise. I joined a nearby gym and didn't really know what I was doing. One of the trainers convinced me to work out with him. He told me my whole diet was wrong and that I needed to definitely eat more to keep my metabolism going. His observation was correct but he was totally off with his suggestions. Some of his breakfast recommendations were high protein smoothies with fruit and peanut butter or giant egg white omelets with a side of oatmeal or whole wheat toast. For lunch it would be turkey or tuna sandwiches (no mayo, of course) on whole grain bread or wraps. Dinner could be pasta or baked potato with grilled chicken or fish and a salad. High protein bars and protein shakes were typical snacks. In addition to water, sports drinks were suggested to replace my electrolytes. He explained that I needed the extra carbs as fuel and that I would burn it all off.

Each session we would work on different body parts. We would focus on biceps and triceps one day, back, chest and shoulders another, then work on legs and butt. All the exercises were done with fairly heavy weights. He wanted to focus on training because that was what he was paid for but he didn't explain how I needed to maintain cardiovascular exercises on my own. I barely biked, did the treadmill, the elliptical or anything that kept my heart rate up. I did practice yoga, but it was Hatha Yoga and there was very little sweating involved.

Six months into my new regimen, guess what the results were? I had thrown on another ten pounds. The trainer explained that it was all muscle. Maybe it was more muscle, but I wasn't a dude that wanted to bulk up! I was really aggravated about how I wasted all this time and money following his program. It's not that the diet was unhealthy or the workouts weren't burning calories. A man would have probably achieved exactly what he wanted. It just wasn't the right protocol for a female who wanted to keep slim. What proved to be effective for his body builder clients was not exactly what I should have been doing. But I still couldn't understand where his methods were flawed for my particular frame.

My need to understand my body's biochemistry led me to study anatomy, physiology and biology in college. I became certified as a Health Coach, received a Bachelor's degree in holistic nutrition along with becoming a licensed massage therapist, certified yoga and group fitness instructor. The next few years I did a lot of experimentation to see which methods would keep me fit as possible. Since I was more holistic and teaching yoga throughout New York City, I thought I had no choice but to be a vegetarian. Any other way of eating would make me a hypocrite. I was also convinced that the diet the trainer put me on had failed because it was too high in animal protein.

I was sure that vegetarian was the healthiest way to go. I used to work a lot of health expos, would spend time at Ashram's and healing circles, and even made friends with Hare Krishnas that would give me some really interesting recipes. Before the term "gluten free" became popularized, I was aware of the benefits of a wheat-free diet. I also eliminated yeast, sugar, and anything processed. I got hugely into beans and lentils and was super creative with the ways I prepared them. Bean burgers were one of my favorites. Then my other staples were brown rice, quinoa, tofu, tempeh, faux meats made from soy and nuts along with steamed vegetables.

The only places where I'd eat were either Indian, macrobiotic, or health food restaurants. Yet to my surprise, I put on another 10 pounds. Now this didn't make sense. Here I am eating a clean diet, no meat, no wheat, no dairy, no sugar and I can't stop blowing up!

All these scenarios of failed attempts could have left me feeling like there was no hope at achieving the body I wanted. I didn't want to be fated to the Eastern European Jewish Bubby frame as I aged because that was encoded in my DNA. I can proudly say now that it doesn't look like I'm going down that road. If anything, people think I'm blessed with good genetics and want to know my secret to staying so slim.

I hope that all my trial and error with the myriad of diets I've been unsuccessful with can prevent you from making the same mistakes. I don't believe anyone is doomed to be fat despite what you consider to be an unfortunate predisposition. Not everyone can be model-skinny, nor should they aspire to be. But my goal is to help you love and take advantage your new body, whether it's in your favorite outfit (the one that's been hiding in the back of your closet), not panic during bathing suit season, and spice up the chemistry with your man - or the guy you've yet to meet!

CHAPTER 1

IDENTIFYING YOUR FAT GIRL HABITS

I can spot these ladies a mile away because I used to make the same dreadful mistakes. The fashion exec at the gym who gulps down a giant smoothie with hemp powder and extra chia seeds after a six mile run, the teacher in the cafeteria who eats only a fruit salad and a diet iced tea for lunch because she's trying to save calories over a regular meal, or the mother at the coffee shop who orders a non-fat gluten-free muffin with a skim latte. It's obvious they think they are making the wiser choice that will ultimately lead to weight loss, but they will never be successful. These are what I call "fat girl habits". I'm saying this in jest - but most people that eat this way end up overweight and can't understand why. I would love to just walk over to them and hand out a business card suggesting a consultation, but it's a touchy subject and no one wants to be embarrassed.

So instead I made this chapter about identifying your fat girl habits in the privacy of your own space. When you look over this questionnaire, don't get discouraged if this all seems too familiar. Actually, it's a good sign because now you know what NOT to do going forward.

Breakfast
1. Do you often skip breakfast?
2. Do you typically have a bowl of cereal?
3. Do you eat gluten free, fat free, or whole grain muffins of any kind?
4. Do you eat whole grain or gluten free bread, bagels, toast, or waffles?

5. Do you drink latte's- even chai latte's of any kind? (non-fat, low-fat or soy)
6. Do you use flavored non-fat non-dairy creamers in your coffee?
7. Do you drink juice other than green? This includes organic and fresh squeezed fruit juice.
8. Do you eat non-fat yogurt that comes pre-mixed with fruit flavoring?
9. Do you drink smoothies with multiple fruits and no protein?
10. Do you eat oatmeal out in a restaurant or from a takeout café?

Lunch
1. Do you often skip lunch?
2. Do you eat sushi – 2 rolls or more?
3. Do you often eat wraps or sandwiches? (even whole wheat)
4. Do you typically have several proteins in your salad? (I.E chicken, mozzarella cheese, and almonds, turkey, egg and chickpeas or tofu, beans and walnuts)
5. Do you apply fat free dressing liberally on your salads?
6. Do you typically get a beverage from the juice bar to drink along with your lunch?
7. Do you snack instead of eating lunch? (Fruit salad with a granola bar, juice, nut milk or coconut water with a gluten free snack, or a bag of organic baby carrots with a small container of hummus)
8. Do you eat rice bowls or noodle dishes of any kind?
9. Do you eat prepared foods from a salad bar or health food store?
10. Do you eat a snack with your lunch? (salad with a bag of pretzels, sandwich with pita chips, A large soup and frozen yogurt)

Dinner
1. Do you usually order an appetizer in addition to eating a full main course?

2. Do you eat large servings of "healthy grains" often with dinner? (quinoa, brown rice, sweet potato)
3. Do you ever get too lazy to cook, so you have 2 bowls of cereal instead?
4. Do you usually cook with sauces, marinades, and dressings?
5. Do you use oils liberally when cooking because they are considered healthy? (olive oil, coconut oil, flax seed oil)
6. Do you drink white wine, beer, champagne, margaritas, cosmos, or other mixed drinks?
7. Do you eat less than 3 hours before going to bed?
8. Do you eat out of a takeout container rather than portion the food onto your plate?
9. Do you favor starchy vegetables over green leafy vegetables? (carrots, corn, peas, lima beans)
10. Do you let yourself get to being starving before you sit down for dinner?

Snacks
1. Do you snack on handfuls of almonds, seeds, or nuts?
2. Do you snack on peanut or almond butter for extra protein?
3. Do you snack on health food products that are bagged or packaged with very little protein? (gluten free pretzels, baked kale chips, dried fruit, rice cakes)
4. Do you snack on gluten free baked goods? (cookies, oat bars, muffins)
5. Do you snack on loose fruit (grapes, cherries, cantaloupe, watermelon) rather than whole fruits such as apples, pears, peaches or plums?
6. Do you snack on fat free frozen yogurt or non-fat sorbet?
7. Do you snack on smoothies with liberal amounts of "Super Foods" and oils? (flax oil, coconut oil, hemp powder, chia seeds, almond, peanut, and cashew butters)

Exercise
1. Do you eat a heavy meal before a workout?
2. Do you exercise close to bed time?
3. Do you go to the juice bar for a smoothie following a workout?
4. Do you use sports drinks, coconut water or juice to replenish instead of water?
5. Do you focus primarily on weight training rather than these cardio exercises? (cycling, running, brisk walking, elliptical)
6. Do you wait 30 seconds or more between reps because the dumbbells are too heavy and you need to rest?
7. Does your cardio workout last less than 45 minutes?
8. Do you practice yoga or Pilates without breaking a sweat?
9. Does your workout only consist of walking to and from the subway station and up the stairs in your non- elevator building?
10. Do you believe you are burning enough calories through adult activities like wild sex and dancing at the club with your girlfriends?

If you answered YES to more than five of these thirty questions, your habits may be stunting your success. The problem is that most people make even more than ten of these mistakes without a clue that they are even issues to begin with. After spending my entire adult life improving my own biology, working with clients, and having tons of skinny obsessed girlfriends, I've become somewhat of a Fat Whisperer, Weight Loss Biohacker, Healthy Detective, and The Doctor House of uncovering what lies beneath the surface.

Without getting defensive, throughout this book I'll explain why many of your efforts were not making a single dent in getting to your goal. I know you can probably back up some of these habits from various blog posts you may find floating around Google. Just because that "expert" may have a nutrition degree, a doctorate, or a personal training certification- take a look at their appearance and their current state of health. Over the years I've crossed paths with several overweight dieticians, personal trainers, physicians, and bestselling authors that didn't look at all like a picture of health. They may be a walking encyclopedia of information but that's not who I would turn to for advice if it hasn't even worked for them in their individual lives. While I have my own health credentials as well, I wouldn't' feel comfortable dispensing advice if I didn't walk the talk and have my own personal success.

I'm asking you to leave your reservations at the door if everything you were previously doing, didn't get you to where you wanted to be. Keep reading- help is on the way!

CHAPTER 2

CHANGE YOUR BELIEFS, CHANGE YOUR BODY

The body we live in is no accident. There still lies a perception, however, that the state of our health, physical capabilities, our weight and the way we look are controlled primarily by our genes. With this primary belief system in place, we may as well just let ourselves go and leave it up to destiny. You may have heard your mother or your friends say while you were growing up, "You're just big-boned." Your older brother and his friends may have teased you about being chubby. Or later in life you may be validated by being told that it's normal to gain weight after college because your metabolism has slowed down. If you have been programmed to believe you are just a victim of bad genetics and aging, then your attempts to take on any diet or exercise plan will resonate into the universe as half ass. Why? Because with that mentality, you don't even trust that you'll be successful. Without conviction or being able to visualize something, it makes it almost impossible to achieve. And if below the surface is just a lot of negative self-talk, even the most stellar program with the best practitioner in the world will most likely not be able to help you.

With an already jaded attitude towards a healthier and thinner body, the sense of commitment is diminished. If you don't see major progress in just a few days or weeks, it's easy to lose motivation and feel like you are killing yourself for nothing. The brain goes back to its old thoughts and programming, resulting in beliefs such as. "This is a waste of time," "I'm not cut out for this lifestyle," "It sucks to be depriving myself," or "I will never look like (whoever your ideal is of beauty) anyway. "

Rather than just flat out quit, you may find yourself taking on bits of healthy behaviors when they are convenient but with no consistency. One day you may have a salad for lunch when the rest of the office orders in pizza; the next day you eat a huge dinner alone at home. Another night you may feel inspired to do a Spin® class but then don't get back to the gym for two more weeks because it's winter and too cold outside. You swear off carbs and eat just protein for three days straight but then after you have no energy and dive into a bowl of pasta followed by ice cream for dessert.

Success doesn't always begin with physical action but instead with mental action. In our mind is where we plant the seeds for growth. In this instance, I'm applying it to weight loss but it holds true for any desire we want to come to fruition.

The brain and the heart are powerful organs that are often neglected when we think about our appearance. They are directly related to how we feel about ourselves starting at a soul level. When the soul is feeling unfulfilled, the heart is sad about our current state of being (i.e., not being thin enough, pretty enough or whatever). The brain will then logically reinforce the negativity with logical reasons why we will never achieve our goals (i.e., becoming more attractive). Sometimes you can't quantify the best success with logic. Doing A + B may not always = C. The body is complex, and while there are formulas for being skinny, don't underestimate the power of your conscious and subconscious mind. It sounds a little hokey but your emotional heart and your logical brain need to be on the same page for the desired outcome to occur. Here are some ways to manifest your perfect body without killing yourself at the gym and following crazy diets.

#1. *Push away Negative Thoughts about your body such as,* "I have a big ass," "My thighs are tree trunks," "My arms are too bulky." Replace these with Positive Thoughts in your head even if it sounds ridiculous to you: "I love my butt in yoga pants," "My thighs are sexy," "My arms are lean and toned."

#2. *Visualize what you want to look like.* Go mentally to the place that would be the ultimate result of all your efforts. If you were a head-turner with an insane figure in high school and are now 30 years old, it's not impossible to look like that again. (I know that firsthand) I gained about 20 pounds in my early 20's with bad habits I was unaware of and always wore black to camouflage it. By the time I hit 26 (and after much visualization), I lost the weight. I didn't know how it would magically happen but as soon as I started seeing the change in my mind, the knowledge and answers to reverse my body appeared. So take that dusty old photo from senior year and hang it on your refrigerator!

If you were always a little overweight and can't paint a mental picture of yourself being any different, use a photo of someone else's body that's closest to your frame. Don't jump ahead to morphing into a small-boned Victoria's Secret model. Instead, pick someone sexy and with curves – think Sophia Vergara or Beyonce') and affix your face on top and post on the fridge.

#3. *Think consciously about how these new changes will impact the quality of life.* The two prior examples were more about feelings on a subconscious level. Now once you've achieved your goal, what will you actually do going forward? What tangible changes can occur? Start thinking about all the things you plan to act on whether it's dating more, going to social events, wearing sexier clothes. These can all be realistic expectations after the next few months.

Some limiting thoughts I beg you to delete are:

#1. *"I'm not beautiful unless I'm thin."* Self-confidence shouldn't be contingent on your size. You can't be excited through the process of getting fitter and healthier if you are self-deprecating. That just creates unnecessary pressure, everyone around you will feel your burden, and you'll probably just quit. Try to enjoy the journey at the pace it comes even if it's slower than your timetable. There are plenty of girls who are objectively thin and pretty but guys don't find them sexy because they are constantly nitpicking and stressing about their appearance. It's a huge turnoff that has nothing to do with aesthetics. If you have a few extra pounds but good energy and can accept yourself at whatever pace your body changes, you will be way more beautiful and desirable than the skinny girl who's insecure.

#2. *"I have to punish myself in order to lose weight."* Who wants to start a program that suggests you now have to basically give up the pleasure of eating, going out to dinner with friends or having a drink on a date because your life will be on hold for whatever duration of this misery? You are not becoming a contestant on The Biggest Loser that has to attend 6 a.m. Bootcamp and get your ass kicked by Jillian Michaels.

This is no punishment but an opportunity. It's your birthright to have a healthy body that's clean, well nourished, and radiant. Putting on makeup, wearing a beautiful dress, and blowing out your hair will all help your case but there is nothing like having a body that moves gracefully, doesn't get bloated, and looks great in a simple t-shirt and jeans. Be a nerd and make this a science project. If you were going to try to create something in chemistry class, you wouldn't use inorganic, synthetic compounds while constructing it. You would work with the resources you had available in nature that would give your new object the greatest chance of surviving with good health. The same holds for your body. Don't think you can fill it up with artificial foods, preservatives and chemicals, and then create a masterpiece. Instead of looking at food as fulfillment, see it in a way that you can ask yourself, "Will this food that I'm ingesting or drink that I'm consuming bring me closer to becoming a work of art to be desired, or a toxin that's going to deplete my energy, confuse my organs, and make me less beautiful than I could be?"

While eating and drinking is a pleasure, overdoing it is a detriment. Duh, you already know that but it goes way beyond being fat or thin. Lack of exercise, eating crappy foods, even overeating so called "health foods" will drain your life force and break your spirit if your body is not happy.

You don't have to tell yourself you can never have a burger, pizza, cookies a glass of champagne or your favorite indulgence. Don't have a guilt trip about skipping the gym if you're tired. That's no way to live and you should enjoy special occasions, weekends and vacations without feeling like a freak around your friends. Yet once you've veered a little, come back to balance (and make that balance a healthy foundation). Not to go off the path so much that your balance point is an unhealthy place (and healthy behaviors are just every now and then).

While people will try to throw you off track as you start to make noticeable progress, don't give in. If someone tried to talk you into smoking crack, would you feel bad by saying no? Of course not because there is a social stigma attached to doing drugs. Even though it probably gives a nice temporary high, I would imagine that you would feel terrible after and end up looking like a crack head with long-term use. More likely than being corrupted by a "drug pusher" is a "food pusher." This could be your mother, your boyfriend, your coworker or anyone with influence. JUST SAY NO. Under their power you may not look as bad as a junky, but you will get fat and it's so not worth it. YOU have to live in your body- not them. Talk to yourself, practice discipline, and every day work to keep your head on straight with your eye on the prize.

CHAPTER 3

STOP STRESSING

I live in the capital of stressful living. While it would be awesome to leave the city myself or tell my clients to just check out and move to a farm or beach town- this is our current reality and we live here for good reason. Most of us need to stick it out (even if temporarily) and can't fully hold our surroundings accountable for our chaos. We have no choice but to try and cope with our day-to-day stress from another perspective. Even if you don't live in Manhattan, everyone has their challenges and the scale of their severity is relative to what they're used to. While it sounds easier said than done, you probably already know that stress can create a lot more damage than just altering your appetite. When you feel overwhelmed, sad or anxiety-ridden, it can seriously screw up your health – including your metabolism. The adrenals may burn out, thyroid function could decline, while cortisol increases and serotonin decreases. The hormones go haywire and the only way to keep going is to shovel in food with sugar and caffeine (i.e., lots of carbs, snacks, coffee and sodas).

The highs and lows that derive from too many refined sugars and carbohydrates that we run to for boosting our serotonin levels have us swinging between temporary pleasure to complete depression. Right after scarfing down one of those stress-induced meals, we feel like we just got our fix. It's like a drug that gives us quick bursts of energy to keep us going or gets us out of a funk. But within just a short amount of time we come down, possibly get irritable, nervous, or even feel guilty for what we just put into our body. Yet, since we never really satisfied our nutritional requirements with all those nutrient void foods, it's likely our bodies will feel hungry before it really should be time to eat again. Although we know they are bad for us, it's an addiction not unlike drugs to reach for those foods again to sustain the high.

Coffee is on the top of my list of things to avoid if you are stressed out. Among most people who have a lot of pressure, coffee is hands down their drug of choice. Even with the antioxidants this beverage can provide, there are more negatives than benefits for someone who needs to chill out. If you're craving a morning boost, you are much better off going for organic green tea. You still get the caffeine and antioxidants you need without the acidity. Green tea also contains a compound called L-Theanine which actually eases anxiety. Already hooked on the habit of knocking back more than one cup of Joe? I've been there and it's certainly easy to do. Just thinking about the delicious smell of the roasted beans, how it gets you going in the morning and keeps you cozy and warm in the winter is so tempting. I feel like I need to go to rehab just talking about it! Multiple cups, however, can spike cortisol levels which increase insulin and inflammation (and ultimately lead to weight gain). Coffee can also trigger anxiety or cause a nervous stomach. Running to the bathroom is the last thing you want on your mind when you have to give a presentation or you're stuck in traffic rushing to work! The other digestive issue triggered by all this caffeine is increased stomach acid which can lead to hunger. Don't forget about insomnia, which may already be an issue with anyone who is heavily stressed.

Now that I bring up insomnia, let's talk a little about sleepless nights. Having puffy eyes and looking cracked out the following day is bad enough but the lack of sleep produces increased levels of the hunger hormone "ghrelin" and decreased levels of the satiety/fullness hormone "leptin". You probably have no desire to work out because you're barely making it through the day as it is. You don't want to perpetuate this seesaw of lousy sleep and using uppers all day to keep you going. When it's finally time to come down and approach bedtime, your wheels are spinning and you're screwed. Ambien™ anyone?

Try to imagine this combination: No exercise, no sleep and you're eating like a ravenous animal on all the wrong foods and snacks possible. This is when it's time to put your foot down, take control, and get it together. Tell yourself that in addition to whatever you are struggling with, you do not want to give power to the guy who broke your heart, the boss who acted like a total asshole, or whatever crummy situation is filling your waking hours. If anything, this is the time when you want to feel your best so you can turn back to that person or situation and say, "Look at me now!"

It's up to you to apply mind over matter if you have any shot at stopping this madness. Instead of going out tonight and bitching with your girlfriends over a highly caloric cocktail, make it your business to get yourself home at a reasonable hour. Shut down your phone and your computer by 10 p.m. because you need to turn off your brain.

Sometimes the things that are stressing us out are out of our control but many times it's more about how we cope with it. When stress gets the best of us and now becomes apparent in our physical well-being, it's time to reflect on our life and make some changes.

Take a look at who is dominant in your inner circle. Is your boss devaluing you or are your hours and responsibilities so overwhelming that they make you not want to get out of bed in the morning? Do you feel unsatisfied or a little dysfunctional in your relationship whether it's with your husband, someone you're dating or someone you are hooking up with and are not even clear if you <u>are</u> dating? Are your girlfriends negative, bitchy, jealous or catty? If so, this could be the root of many of your bad habits. You have to get a little selfish. The girl inside you that wants to be liked or please everyone may need to take a different course of action.

You are going to do two things here; specifically, a cleansing of house both inner and outer. For all those unwanted people who bring you aggravation, slowly start being unavailable. You don't have to unfriend them from Facebook and make it obvious that you are pulling away because this will cause more stress and drama on its own. Instead, just be "busy" and eventually they will get the message.

As for your employer, you may not have the leisure of quitting but you don't have to let your job define you, either. If you are doing the best you can, go ahead and let your boss rant. Some people of authority just like to throw around their power because work is the only place they feel important. Maybe they have marital problems or their kids drive them nuts and they subsequently take out that displaced aggression on you. Who knows what is going on in their private lives which makes them difficult to deal with! See what happens if you take it on as a personal experiment to not be reactive and not give their pressures or criticisms so much meaning. Nothing is worth the cost of your health. If you're not doing something you're passionate about and not running your own business anyway, stay cool and use that frustration as a catalyst to create a new opportunity with another company or your own thing. Life is too short to spend at least eight hours a day doing something that makes you unhappy.

When you're not fixated on work or responsibilities, don't allow eating and drinking always to be your "go to" activities for fun. If that's really how you prefer to unwind, then save it for the weekends. But for now on Monday through Thursday, that should be YOU time. If you suffer from F.O.M.O (fear of missing out) on an event or something social, you're not. If you're running yourself ragged, stressed, possibly not sleeping and are now gaining weight as a result, your health and your appearance just go downhill as you age. And trust me, as you get into your late 30's 40's and 50's, that will just lead to more stress and depression. It's better to be the hot, in-shape woman that only makes an occasional appearance because she's too busy getting her "exercise on" than the woman who's out in the scene looking a little frumpy and tired.

The best option to de-stress in your free time would obviously be to get yourself to do something physical but not too late in the evening since that can cause insomnia as well. Sometimes you need to blow off evening plans in order to be fresh for a 6 a.m. workout the next day. Getting to the gym, taking a kickboxing class, going for a run, doing yoga, etc. are great for a number of reasons. They all help you to pump up your endorphins, release negative energy, and you'll will start your day or come home in a better mood with the added benefit of sleeping better.

Truth be told, not everyone likes to exercise. I have several clients I work with that have gym memberships and have never used the facility. For whatever reason, they can't get the motivation going. If you are one of these people, I hope that's something you can work on. And if your metabolism is already slow from lack of physical fitness, then not being conscious of your diet will be even more detrimental.

The second best thing you can do is take a class in the evening or make plans that don't revolve around food as entertainment. Take an art class, learn a new language or explore your spirituality. Just simply getting your mind out of a negative place and not focusing on your worries will ease your stress levels as well as put things in a fresh perspective.

As you start eliminating the wrong people from your life and focusing on things that bring fulfillment, you will be in a better emotional place to change your eating habits. You won't need to look at food for comfort. You will find that you are eating because you are truly hungry and not out of stress or nervousness. Eating without being harried, peer pressured or persuaded from the alcohol talking will allow you to eat in a more mindful manner. Watch how your body naturally begins to desire foods like fruits and vegetables over anything junky. When you reduce the stress in your life, a clean diet will only become a side effect. The benefits will spill over to every area in your life improving health, relationships, and patience to not make big deals out of things that were not worth stressing over in the first place!

CHAPTER 4

WHAT'S IN A PORTION?

Have you ever noticed women who snack on a little junk food whenever they feel like it without a second thought, eat moderately, and yet seem to have fewer weight issues than someone who never breaks down for a piece of cake or a bagel, constantly diets, but gorges on health foods. It kind of sounds like the European verses American mentality, doesn't it? The French can have a three-course meal with no thought of carb counting or skipping dessert because everything is properly portioned. Leave it to a fat American to polish off a giant salad at The Cheesecake Factory that can feed an entire table of those chic and skinny women!

Maimonides, one of the greatest physicians of all time, often spoke about overeating and why we shouldn't do it. To this day his theories on health from thousands of years ago still hold up. In his ancient writings, he states that overeating even "good foods" is unhealthy. Proclaimed Superfoods like kale, wild salmon, raw almonds or organic berries can be awesome. Yet, there is a limit to what the body can handle and that means there are no free foods. In the same way, water is essential. But did you know that drinking too much of it can kill us? Likewise, sex is necessary for relationships to flourish and to experience pleasure, but in excess it's depleting. If we follow the natural laws of the universe, it's clear that food is no different.

Digestion comes into play each time we eat and we can't overburden our system if we want it to do a good job. People who follow low-carb diets fall victim to this all the time. Let's say there's a catered event that is serving wraps, or you are at a deli-style restaurant that has an open faced sandwich. If you throw out the wrap or bread but eat 10 ounces of meat or protein inside and have it with a salad, it sounds like an okay idea. Yet in truth it's a giant portion! While I'm not a fan of most commercial breads because they are usually very processed, it's better to have a little bite of the sandwich and a normal-sized portion than an overflowing salad with too many ingredients – including gobs of dressing!

First you should familiarize yourself with what a portion looks like. Typically when you eat in a restaurant, a meal is at least a double portion. Before you take your first bite, get into the habit of slicing your food in half and pushing the remainder to the side. If you are on a date or a business meeting and trying not to look strange, you can do this discreetly.

If you also had an appetizer, visualize the amount of food you just ate prior to your dinner sitting next to your entrée. That should help you calculate how much more you should be taking in. Then add on any bread. Some people make the mistake of eating a regular amount but they eat a few slices of bread beforehand and don't really think that counts. Take note that even though you may have had fish and vegetables for dinner, with the bread included it's about the equivalent of eating a slice or two of pizza. Probably even worse since pizza just has sauce and cheese. You are now adding on fish and an entire serving of vegetables that was probably sautéed in oil.

While I'm not advocating Weight Watchers™, it was on the right track when it came up with the Point System. It's about budgeting like we all do when working through our expenses. If you know you have to pay for your rent, cell phone, car insurance, gas or public transportation, those are fixed costs you can't get around. You do, however, have some control over how many times you do dinner or drinks with the girls, go shopping for new bags/shoes or get a mani/pedi /blowout. These nonessentials that are social or make us feel pretty have to be well thought out unless we have an expendable bank account, generous husband or a sugar daddy. I personally allot myself one manicure and blowout per week. If for some reason it rains and I get frizzy or I chip a nail in a yoga class, then it's on me to fix it up myself at home. I've also trained myself to only take taxis at night and public transportation or walking during the day. Dinners and drinks with friends in NY add up so I have to be conscious of making other plans that don't require spending money.

We have to look at our eating habits like our budget. I like to call this our Food Budget. Eating something for breakfast, lunch and dinner are like those fixed costs we can't get around. We need to eat to function, yet we need to account for all the extras. If we want to have a few glasses of wine per week and a dessert, that's like our mani/pedi/blowout budget. But if we go beyond that with eating full-sized entrees at dinner and raiding the bread basket, it's as if we've spent anything we have left on cab fare and now we can't afford our rent.

To go back to basics, let's get clear on how to visualize a portion.

Protein A serving of protein should be around 4-6 ounces. Four ounces is roughly the size of your fist. The next time you're eating a piece of fish, meat, or poultry, have that in mind. You should be conscious of not eating more than a fist and a half of any of these main foods at a time.

Fats Healthy fats such as olive oil, flax oil, coconut oil or almond butter can be eaten daily but not poured liberally because the fat and calorie content will add up. Each tablespoon is around 100 calories and contains over 10 grams of fat. Without paying attention, you can easily rack up 300-400 calories and 30-40 grams of fat with these oils or butters alone without even calculating the additional ingredients in your meal. Use an actual tablespoon to serve yourself and follow the same guidelines with high-calorie condiments such as mayonnaise, salad dressing or tahini. So although salads and vegetables are healthy, a giant portion will most likely not be eaten raw. Think about how much dressing or oil is required to make an overflowing bowl of kale taste good. Is it 4, 5, 6 tablespoons? Maybe more?

Carbohydrates While you don't have to be too conscious about the carbohydrates in most vegetables (especially the green leafy ones), healthy starches like rice, quinoa, sweet potato, butternut squash, amaranth and non-gluten containing grains still need to be portioned. A half cup is recommended for a modest serving and one cup if you are eating it early in the day, worked out, or just feel really hungry, since these are all high in carbohydrates. Visualize a baseball as one cup and then determine if you should divide that in half.

When eating fruit, stick to whole fruit which is much easier to portion out. Try to avoid loose grapes, chopped watermelon, papaya, mango, etc. (although they have many vitamins and nutrients). It's very easy to sit in bed watching a movie while eating a pound of any of these fruits in a large bowl as if they were popcorn. Without paying attention, you could easily eat a few hundred calories with hefty amounts of fructose and carbohydrates. Having an organic peach, pear, apple or orange (when in season) will prevent you from overeating. To make it last longer you can cut it into small slices and add a few raw nuts to make it more satisfying, yet you'll know when it's time to stop. Berries happen to be loose fruits which are the exception, but better not to have them as a standalone snack. A half cup is too small of a serving size to generally be satisfying. Berries are great, though, when combined with yogurt, a smoothie or as a side to your morning omelet.

Think about the way your normally eat when you go out. If you are at an Asian restaurant and decide to have a spicy tuna roll as a starter, then sea bass with rice and vegetables as a main course - your food choices aren't bad. But if your goal is to have 4-6 ounces of protein, the tuna in your appetizer may be 3-4 ounces and the rice could already be equivalent to one cup. You don't have to do too much math here, but if you plan to now eat your entire entrée, you are probably eating several portions more than you need. You should reflect on the fact you've already allotted calories, fats, proteins and carbohydrates to the tuna roll. To stay within your Food Budget, only eat about half your sea bass with all the vegetables you want but push the rice to the side.

The same goes for eating at an event whether it's a charity, holiday party, wedding, christening or bar mitzvah. If you found yourself at the carving station before sitting down for the meal, those foods count. When it's time for your entrée, remember you have to subtract that from your dinner. It's fine to have half the protein (chicken, fish or steak) with a nice serving of vegetables, but no rice, potato, pasta or grain.

While it's important to be a lady and observe proper etiquette, I often suggest using improper dishes and utensils to avoid overeating. These are three takeaways that can be useful for life.

1. *Only apply this takeaway if you're with familiar company:* When in a restaurant, you can ask the waiter for an extra plate (which is usually smaller than your dinner plate). Portion your serving onto the small dish leaving the remainder on the large plate. After you've finished, do not go back to your original plate for seconds.
2. Eat on smaller dishes at home that look more like saucers than Frisbees. Your food should look balanced, not piled up to the ceiling or spilling off the edges.
3. Get into the habit of using tea cups and teaspoons. Soups, cereals, oatmeal or any breakfast grain are generally ½ to 1 cup serving.

You can visualize your portion just by knowing you are eating out of an actual cup. Most of the time people use a bowl (which is equivalent to several servings). Instead of a tablespoon, use a teaspoon for smaller bites. The first time you do this in front of your new boyfriend after a sleepover he may think you're totally nuts but who cares!

Knowing your portions allows you to enjoy going out for dinner, being social, going on vacation and never having to worry about getting fat. While there are healthier choices than others, sometimes you want to splurge on food that's not so ideal. I promise if you do that every now and then (but in small doses), it won't even make a dent in your weight. That's how French women can eat a piece of fattening cheese or a few bites of decadent chocolate without gaining an ounce. It's all about knowing how to be mindful of not going overboard. When you drink alcohol, there are clues to let you know you're getting bombed and need to cut back. People around you will probably even tell you to slow down. Unless you have a sensitive stomach, it's easy to be unconscious about your food intake. No one is going to call you out on eating too much. Don't feel compelled to whip out your calculator, but please reflect on your Food Budget prior to each bite.

CHAPTER 5

DON'T WASTE A WORKOUT

If you are religious about your workouts - yet still don't have the body you want- there a number of things to consider. Exercising is beneficial but it's not as simple as just dedicating an hour a day to something physical. What are you doing in that hour? Exercise also will provide little value if you're kind of like "Well, what I eat is not really a big deal because I'll burn it off anyway." Think about your routine and then review the following questions.

1. Are you getting in enough cardio? Do you use the elliptical, bike or treadmill or usually take classes?
2. Do you use free weights? If so, do you rest between sets?
3. Do you skip cardio all together and solely use machines for weight-bearing exercises?
4. What time of day do you work out?
5. Do you usually eat a full meal before a workout?
6. What do you eat or drink following a workout?

We'll get back to these questions shortly, but although you may disagree with me I believe that taking off weight is 80% diet and 20% exercise. I have seen countless cases where women have come to me to lose weight and their chief complaint is, "I work out all the time but just bulk up". So let's dissect why this may be happening.

Rule #1. *A workout will not promote weight loss without cardio.* A bare minimum 30-45 minutes of cycling, brisk walking, elliptical, or spinning is required at least 3-4 times a week to see any results. Men have a different training routine because they want to build size and muscle. For them, short intense exercises provide the best results. Since our anatomy is very different, I wouldn't suggest going to the gym with your boyfriend and following his routine.

As a female, the priority is usually to slim down and lean out. Yoga, Pilates and weight training are all encouraged, but if the goal is losing weight they should be in addition to your cardio workouts. If you are doing a super vigorous practice such as Astanga or Vinyasa yoga, that is the exception. As a former group fitness instructor at Equinox Fitness, The Sports Club LA, The Reebok Sports Club and Exhale Spa, I can appreciate a talented instructor or personal trainer. Yet set aside time for vigorous cardio (cycling, running, brisk walking, elliptical) as often as possible. If you have never worked out before, it's advised to start off slow and build up your tolerance. Rather than 30-45 minutes on day one, start with 15 minutes cardio. Keep adding on five additional minutes each week, although you don't need to go past an hour which is plenty. Just try to boost up your cardio to at least 3 days per week.

Rule #2. *Lifting weights should NOT make you gain weight.* If you've been under the influence of a trainer that wants you to keep increasing the amount of weight you are lifting, that may not be necessary. Weight-bearing exercises will actually contribute to weight loss when done in addition to consistent cardio. It speeds up your metabolic rate and will lead to burning additional calories even when you are not active. The best way to lift weights is by focusing on free weights. Rather than do a set of only 10 bicep curls with two 12 pound weights, use lighter weights (5, 8 or 10 pounds) and do a set of 30 bicep curls. Instead of taking your normal 30-60 second rest in between sets, use that time to hop right into another exercise such as lunges. Then as soon as you finish a set of 30 lunges with light weights, jump right back into your bicep curls. This type of high rep, low weight workout will lean you out while giving beautiful definition to your body parts. When using the machines, it's easy to rely on them for support. Free weights require more balance and core strength which is sometimes harder, yet will lead to more aesthetic results.

Rule # 3. *When you work out matters.* One of the worst times to work out is right after you've eaten a main meal (except for breakfast) since that's a light meal to begin with. You have to time your workouts and here's why. Let's say you eat a big lunch at noon and then go for a workout at 1 p.m. Despite the fact you probably won't have fully digested your food, you will also work up an appetite too early. When you are done around 2 or 3 p.m., you will be ready for another meal. A protein shake may hold you over if you plan to have dinner by 5 p.m., but who eats dinner at that time? Maybe your grandparents in Boca Raton. Since we are more social in other parts of the world, dinner is not until 7, 8 or 9 p.m. and that will create a problem. You don't want to go into a dinner meal being ravenous. You'll end up overeating and that negates any benefit from your time at the gym.

You also don't want to have dinner and then go to the gym after 8 p.m. This is for the same reason of eating way too late at night. If you get home around 9:30-10 p.m. and your workout was worthwhile, once again you will be very hungry. Now if you are disciplined and can have Greek yogurt, some grilled chicken breast or turkey slices then it's not a problem. Yet most people can't stop with just a light snack and end up overeating right before bed. It's one of the sure ways to keep on the weight despite how many calories you may have just burned. The other problem with late workouts is that they can be over-stimulating and not good when trying to unwind and get in a good night's sleep – which is another key to weight loss.

The best thing is to eat very light before a workout, enough food to give you energy but not something that qualifies as an actual meal. In fact, a lot of athletes and competitive body builders who want to look shredded often skip meals prior to a workout for better results. Some studies have shown that pre-workout fasting helps metabolism and prevents insulin resistance. With that being said, you shouldn't exercise if you are feeling extremely hungry or low energy. Personally, my blood sugar tends to drop when I don't eat enough and I would probably pass out without a snack so you need to know your body. I don't need much; just a little bit of protein like a hard-boiled egg or a scoop of protein powder does the job without overeating.

Getting into the habit of planning workouts around meal times is the way to not eat double meals. For example, having breakfast at 6:30 a.m. and having a second breakfast at 9 a.m. after cycling, or eating lunch at noon- going for a run an hour later and having another lunch around 3 p.m., or lastly (which is the worst) eating dinner at 6 p.m., taking a yoga class at 8 p.m., then coming home at 9:30-10 p.m. and eating once more - which will end up calorically being a second dinner when all is said and done.

Since we discussed eating light prior to a workout, that is the way to save calories. Below is an example on how to time your exercise.

For Early Bird Workouts
6 a.m. (Exercise Time): Go to the gym on an empty stomach. If you need a little something, have a scoop of protein powder in water or one hard-boiled egg.

8-8:30 a.m. (Meal Time): This should have given you sufficient time to exercise, shower and blow your hair. Now you can have a regular breakfast like an omelet, Greek Yogurt, oatmeal or something healthy.

For Lunch Time Workouts

12:30 p.m. (Exercise Time): Have a light protein bar, shake, yogurt or snack that is high in protein and 200 calories or under. *Do not eat lunch beforehand* – hold off until your workout is finished.

2-2:30 p.m. (Meal Time): Eat a lunch high in protein - fish or poultry is great or alternatively tofu, tempeh or beans if you are a vegetarian. Make sure to have a lot of vegetables since you've worked up an appetite. If you are craving more carbohydrates, stick to non-glutenous grains such as quinoa and brown rice or starches like yams, butternut squash and sweet potato. Since you got a late start, this should hold you over until dinner without snacking.

For Late Afternoon Workouts

4 -5 p.m. (Exercise Time): This is actually the ideal time to exercise if you are not a morning person. Unfortunately, it's a little tricky if you have a full time job, yet doable on the weekends. If you eat lunch around 12 or 1 p.m., you still have enough time to digest and will possibly be full enough to jump right into a workout or have just a light snack before or after that will hold you over comfortably for dinner.

7-7:30p.m. (Meal Time): If you work out at 4 p.m., I recommend exercising first, then having a snack around 5:30 p.m., which would leave you the perfect appetite for a 7:30 p.m. dinner. If you are doing a 5 p.m. workout, have the snack right before. By the time you finish, shower and clean up for dinner, it will be 7 or 7:30 p.m. as well.

For Evening Workouts – *Don't Start Too Late*

6-7 p.m. (Exercise Time): Exercising at this hour is more practical for the working world. Yet I wouldn't suggest going to the gym after this time.

8-8:30 (Meal Time): Make sure to have a snack beforehand and try to have dinner by 8:30 p.m. at the latest. Since dinner is now so close to bedtime, you have to be careful of your carbs in the evening. You probably already know that foods like bread, pasta, rice, potatoes and beans are high in calories and carbohydrates. These foods also usually don't taste good plain. Once you've added oil, cheese, condiments, etc., you will have way too much sugar and fat circulating in your bloodstream that will not help your waist line. Regardless or not of whether you've worked out, you will not have the time to burn them off. So although you just did this killer workout, you would have been just as good (even better actually) skipping the heavy exercise and doing some stretching at home followed by a lighter dinner at an earlier hour.

While not all starches are bad, you need to be aware of your quantities at this hour. If you have slow burning carbs such as quinoa, brown rice, yams, or sweet potato, have only a half portion. Add it as an ingredient to your salad or if it's a side dish, eat only ½ cup. Following evening workouts should be a meal that contains a lean protein with clean vegetables. (Not Chinese takeout on the way home that's dripping in sauce.) Chicken, turkey, fish, tofu, cottage cheese – you get the picture - with either a salad or broccoli, spinach, asparagus, kale, cauliflower, beets, eggplant cooked either steamed or in olive oil. You don't have to be so portion conscious if you watch your potatoes and grains. The only issue with this style of eating takes preparation. It's easier to find pizza, pasta or a wrap much more quickly than chopping up a salad and roasting some fish and vegetables. Have a plan before you exercise so you're not left replacing the calories you just burned on the bread that came with your delivery order.

And before you obsess too much about how you didn't work out hard enough or if you totally didn't work out at all, DON'T. It really comes down to what you put in your mouth. It's better to have healthy habits like taking the stairs when possible, not looking for the closest parking spot and accepting the 20 yard walk or just simply not sitting on your butt all day, combined with a really well managed diet than exercising heavily and eating all wrong. When I travel I almost always lose weight and don't work out. It's because I'm cautious about unfamiliar food so I eat light and also walk around leisurely seeing the sights. Spending two or three weeks out of the gym is not problematic, yet I miss the way it makes me feel. Being physically fit is an important goal and it's never too late to get there. Yet before you commit to becoming an athlete to master your perfect body, sometimes less is more.

CHAPTER 6

YOU ARE NOT A SUMO WRESTLER

In 2004 I had a great job working in a holistic medical center in Manhattan. Without much notice, the doctor had to shut down the practice and everyone was let go. Besides losing income, the process of sending out resumes and looking for a new position was obviously stressful. My next door neighbor happened to be in the entertainment field and came to me about a job opening she heard of that paid pretty well. I thought it could be a fun change even if temporary. When you're young it's much easier to be adventurous even if you have no clue what you're doing or if it's maybe completely out of your realm. Your ego doesn't get too bruised if you screw up.

The position was for an executive assistant to the CEO of The World Sumo Challenge. "Huh, what the hell is that?" was the first thing that came to mind. She explained that sumo wrestlers would be flown in from all over the world to participate in this competition at Madison Square Garden. My responsibilities were to manage their hotel bookings, book their flights (which would be two first class seats per person since they couldn't fit into one chair), and take them to weigh-ins, press conferences, and TV appearances. As crazy as it sounded, there was also a part of me that thought it was kind of cool and would make for good cocktail party conversation for the rest of my life.

I became somewhat of a sumo wrangler managing these enormous Japanese, Mongolian and Hawaiian guys. During that time I learned a lot about their eating habits. Just like any competitive athlete, sumo wrestlers need to maintain their weight. There is a formula involved and it's surprisingly not just eating high calorie foods all day long. Actually, their diet may be quite the opposite of what you'd expect! Rather than feed themselves every hour, they often skip breakfast and eat only one to two very large meals a day. Despite their heavy physical activity and great feats of strength, it's not enough to undo the effects of food bombing - not to mention all the alcohol in one sitting. When a female eats in this fashion, it's bad news. So even if you are training for an Iron Woman competition, if you eat and drink without abandon (even just one meal a day), your physical efforts won't save you.

Many women are scared to snack for fear that they are eating too much throughout the day.

Overweight women are especially self-conscious about snacking. When I see them during a consultation, they almost applaud themselves for not having breakfast, maybe skipping lunch again or having something light like a half a sandwich or a carby oat bar or muffin with a juice, latte or chai, and then having a regular dinner. But the question is, "what are they eating for dinner?"

Think about how children eat. Their parents make sure they have a little breakfast, they run around and play, then have a little snack before lunch. They eat a little of whatever is on their plate, run around some more and probably have a snack later. Then they have a little dinner and usually leave the table before finishing. Before bed they may have a small piece of something sweet and that's it. Children don't tend to gorge themselves at any meal because their parents are on top of them having something satisfying and nutritious every few hours. Although we may not have the metabolism of a 10 year old, the way in which they eat and move is keeping them like skinny string beans.

So let's do the math here. This is an example of someone who grazes on healthy foods throughout the day:

Breakfast Two scrambled eggs with spinach and mushrooms. Side of sliced tomato (240 calories)
Mid-Morning Snack One individual serving Low-Fat Greek yogurt (150 calories)
Lunch Grilled chicken salad with cooked yellow and green squash, beets, and red peppers. Side of quinoa (500 calories)
Mid-Afternoon Snack 12 raw almonds and an apple (170 calories)
Dinner Baked salmon with side of grilled asparagus and small salad of lettuce, cucumbers, avocado and tomato. Olive oil dressing (550 calories)
One glass of wine or two vodka/club sodas (110 calories)
One small piece of hard cheese with two organic dark chocolate squares (170 calories)
Total calories = 1780

By grazing throughout the day, your metabolism stays revved, keeps you burning calories, and stabilizes your blood sugar. You also know another meal is coming in a few hours so you don't need to chow all in one serving. This is the worst at dinnertime and, interestingly, another sumo habit. They have a heavy meal at night and then go to sleep. If you eat late and don't have a chance to burn those calories off, (especially all those carbohydrates), they will turn into sugar and get stored as fat. This is the main reason why I don't recommend exercising late at night, since you will go home hungry and typically overeat at the wrong hour.

The following example is of someone who doesn't really eat during the day but saves it up for later:

Breakfast Large latte with skim milk and Splenda™. (180 calories)
There is no lunch - only a small snack based on the rationale it's better to skip the meal
4 p.m. Break Coffee with a muffin or "natural" snack like pretzels and a small container of hummus (500-700 calories) Even if you consumed less calories, this type of meal is not nutrient dense, high in carbohydrates and will still leave you feeling hungry.
Dinner = Starvation
You have a roll because you are starving. Then you may have another and this one has a little butter or olive oil. Trying to eat healthy, you start off with a plate of salad. This is followed by grilled chicken with vegetables and rice. After finishing your meal, you still don't feel satisfied so you go back to get seconds. Now you've just had a double portion of food and carb loaded on rice right before bed. Trying to practice portion control if you are starving doesn't work very well! (1900 calories)

If you are not conscious of drinking, it's easy to have two glasses of wine without a second thought (220 calories)
Evening Snack Bowl of fruit (grapes, cantaloupe, watermelon or whatever is in season). You would assume fruit is healthy - right? (200-300 calories)
Total calories = 2120-2420

Now some women may need to have this amount of calories in their diet if they are physically active. What you need to know, however, is that a day of eating is not based on the total number of calories consumed but, rather, the quality and nutritional breakdown.

Someone who eats 2,300 calories (coming from nutrient dense foods) distributed over a 14-hour period will have a faster metabolism than a person who eats the same amount all in one meal plus a snack that holds no nutritional value. Ideally, you want to train your body to burn calories faster. The way you do this is by exercising (but not solely) as well as eating frequent meals. Everyone has heard at one time or another that if you wait long periods between meals, the body is unsure when it will eat again so it holds on to the calories in the last meal it consumed. Sumo wrestlers understand this concept. So before you pat yourself on the back for going an entire day with barely eating aside from your one meal, I guarantee that you are doing yourself a huge disservice.

This pattern of eating also leads to blood sugar imbalances. When your sugar gets too low, you crave starchy foods or sugar to bring yourself back to equilibrium – which is only temporary. Someone who eats every few hours may be fine eating a diet lower in starchy carbohydrates and excess grains (which contribute to weight gain) because their sugar levels are balanced and they are not depleted. On the other hand, those who wait until they are ravenous will end up not having self-control by dinnertime. They will likely need to eat double or triple the amount of food compared to the person who didn't skip meals. Additionally, they are more likely to want a more filling evening snack.

While fruit seems healthy as a snack choice, too much of it can be high in sugar and carbohydrates to have in the evening. Although a small piece of cheese and square of chocolate contains more fat, it's actually more satisfying and you can stop there without overdoing it. Unfortunately, if you are feeling hungry following dinner, this kind of light snack or a single pear or apple won't satiate you. Only a giant bowl of fruit will!

Even if you are busy at work, have children to take care of, or just don't feel hungry during the day, don't let that be an excuse for not eating. As the sumo wrestlers have pointed out, saving it up for later is a major fat girl habit.

CHAPTER 7

PROTEIN IS A GIRL'S BEST FRIEND

"I'm always hungry." "I have so many cravings." "I'm a carbaholic." "When I eat healthy I'm never satisfied." These are things I hear all the time from clients. Most people believe the notion that losing weight or staying thin has to be painful and that hunger comes with the territory. When trying to diet, it's common to shy away from high-protein foods because they provoke a fear associated with weight gain and because they appear as heavy. While plant foods such as beans, legumes and nuts have some protein as well as dairy, the best sources come from wild-caught fish, free-range eggs, grass-fed meats, and organic poultry.

Let's talk a little about protein and why we need it. Proteins are made up of building blocks called amino acids. Protein helps us get those beautifully defined muscles, prevents brittle hair, skin, and nails, strengthens our bones, and is needed for proper hormone function. Two hormones that are affected by our diets and the amount of protein we eat are insulin and leptin and they work in tandem. Our bodies use insulin to process carbohydrates and regulate blood sugar. Yet when we live on high-carbohydrate, high-sugar, low-protein diets, we can produce too much insulin. Not only does that put us at risk for diabetes down the road, but too much insulin also increases the storage of fat in our fat cells. So essentially we can eat a "low-fat" or "fat-free" Standard American Diet heavy on grains or starches but it will still make us gain more weight than a high-protein diet which in comparison contains more fat (although it does not trigger the same kind of insulin response). The other hormone called leptin comes from the Greek word "leptos" which means "thin." Increased leptin leads to a speedier metabolism and decreased hunger. Eating protein helps us produce more leptin which signals the brain to make us feel full on fewer calories. When we take protein out of the equation, over time we can set ourselves up for insulin and leptin resistance; both are associated with obesity.

The dieting mentality is to eat as little and light as possible. Diet pills and fat burners are often used to help the process along, but ultimately they don't work and are dangerous with long-term use. There are also a million natural supplements that supposedly speed up your metabolism, prevent the absorption of carbohydrates, etc. but even that approach won't do much once you go back to eating the wrong foods. Eating light is a good idea, although it doesn't have to be with the exclusion of protein. I'm not advocating greasy bacon cheeseburgers with no bun but, rather, eating high-quality lean proteins at meal times or as a snack.

What happens when you skimp on protein is that it takes more calories and larger portions to feel satisfied. For example; let's compare a breakfast of sugar-free cereal and skim milk verses a spinach omelet. The cereal may seem like the more appropriate choice but let's see how it stacks up side by side.

- Two eggs and raw spinach cooked in non-fat olive oil spray = approximately 200 calories and 15 grams of protein.
- Sugar-free cereal may be 100 calories per serving, and 45 calories when the skim milk is added. Although if you read the label, cereal servings are only ½ cup. I don't know anyone who eats that small

of a portion except toddlers! So if you consider a bowl of cereal and skim milk, now multiply that number by 3.

Not only do the eggs provide more nutrition than the cereal, they also win in terms of fewer calories. Eggs will not spike insulin levels (which make us store fat), and keep us fuller longer without looking at the clock by our desk all morning waiting for our lunch break to roll around.

Now I get it if you don't have time to whip up an omelet or you're not a fan of quick hard-boiled eggs. Other high-protein breakfasts are low-fat Greek yogurt, a high-quality protein powder with water (not milk), or even a single serving packet of organic oatmeal with nuts. Since we tend to overeat portions of cereal and oatmeal when it's a self serving, pre-packaged portions keep us in check. Yet the constitution of oatmeal is primarily carbohydrates. As discussed, to prevent an insulin spike, add some raw almonds to your oatmeal. The extra protein in addition to the fiber in the oatmeal will keep you fuller longer. For even better blood sugar control, sprinkle in some cinnamon which has been studied to be a valuable spice.

Lunch time and dinner meals should be balanced. For weight loss, I tell my clients to make their plate 70% green. That means filling it with mostly green leafy vegetables or non-starchy salad ingredients. The other 30% can be a combination of protein and healthy fat. For example, a dish of wild salmon with spinach salad, sliced avocado and a side of asparagus drizzled in olive oil. Or organic turkey breast with kale salad and Brussels sprouts lightly dressed in garlic and oil. Adding low-glycemic and gluten-free carbohydrates such as quinoa, sweet potato, brown rice and starchy vegetables (beets, turnips, corn, squash) are okay in small quantities, but should not be the sum of your meal. Avoid extremely high-carbohydrate meals such as a brown rice bowl with beans/lentils or a plate of quinoa (although both high in protein); they will make you gain weight.

If you noticed, I didn't say to eat protein on its own. Vegetables should be eaten with your meals for several reasons. Two popular diets that advocate a high-protein meal without fruits or vegetables are The Atkins Diet™ and The Dukan Diet™. The reason fruits and vegetables are to be avoided on those programs is because of their carbohydrate content. Even though it's still low, not having any carbohydrates and having very low insulin levels over a period of time can bring the body to a state of "ketosis." Ketosis occurs when you don't have enough sugar (glucose) for energy, so your body breaks down stored fat, causing ketones to build up in your body. It's true that you will most likely lose weight initially on either one of these plans, but it's not healthy and there can be side effects. The issue is that long-term diets like these are highly acidic. In general, high-protein foods are acid-forming. The good news is we can offset the acidity by eating alkaline foods. Fruits and vegetables contain these alkalizing properties and keep the body in that proper acid/alkaline balance.

If you compare the meals I just mentioned – salmon or turkey with vegetables verses a rice or quinoa bowl – you'll see why the low-carb, higher quality protein meal is better for weight loss. The high-protein, low-carb vegetable dishes are around 4-500 calories, contain 20-30 grams of fat, 20-30 grams of protein and are typically under 15 grams of carbohydrates. The protein bowls with rice or quinoa come in to be close in terms of protein, yet are higher calorically and the worst part is their carbohydrate content. Sometimes these bowls can be over 100 grams of carbohydrates, causing a spike in our blood sugar and ultimately bulking us up.

When sticking to high-protein, staying low-carb is the way to go when you want to lose weight. For snacking purposes or as a breakfast alternative – here's the skinny on protein shakes and bars.

Whey protein can be a great choice since it's a complete protein, helps to enhance body composition, suppress appetite, and there are many brands relatively low in calories while high in protein. You can stay full for hours on a 150 calorie shake or whey protein bar under 200 calories. Still some people experience side effects if they are lactose intolerant, and even those who aren't may feel bloating. Many whey proteins brands remove the lactose and it will let you know on the label. Some whey proteins also contain artificial sweeteners, so do a background check on the manufacturer.

Soy Protein is a complete protein, usually dairy-free, yet can still cause some gas and bloating since not everyone can digest soy. There are a lot of really delicious brands of soy proteins found in bars or shakes. Soy protein is typically low in calories and carbohydrates. Just be advised that there is some controversy that soy protein powders contain *phytoestrogens* which mimic estrogen – and there is a link between high estrogen and cancer risk. While this is not a problem for everyone, if you suffer from Poly Cystic Ovary Syndrome (PCOS) – which has a relationship to Estrogen Dominance – you should probably use an alternate protein source. Otherwise, soy protein shouldn't have an entirely bad rap. Studies have linked soy protein to lowering cholesterol, reducing osteoporosis and heart disease. If you choose to go the soy protein route, it's best to alternate between soy and another protein source and to limit to 2-3 shakes or bars a week.

Rice Protein is one of the least allergenic proteins for people with soy and dairy sensitivities. It's a little higher in carbohydrates than whey or soy protein and it's not a complete protein unless it's paired with another protein to complete the amino acid profile. For that reason you may not find it as filling. Still, it's easily digested and is a good alternative for someone who can't tolerate other options. Adding an ingredient like chia seeds (a complete protein) will help make this a more nutritionally balanced shake. If you're eating a rice protein bar, look for ones that contain other proteins besides rice alone.

Pea Protein is another easily digested protein that is usually safe for people with certain food intolerances. Similar to rice protein, it's incomplete and should be mixed with another protein to contain all the necessary amino acids. Just keep in mind, though, that the more proteins you add to one shake, the higher in calories it will be. Very few bars are being made with pea protein these days but they are most likely on the way!

Hemp Protein is almost a complete protein and has the advantage of being high in fiber and contains Omega-6 essential fatty acids. Just be cautious about the brand of hemp protein you choose. They are not all created equal and some hemp proteins are extremely caloric!

Besides high-protein meals and snacks, protein will save you after a night out without the weight gain. Partying until 4 a.m. will almost ensure you work up an appetite. If you are pulled into a late night diner or cafe and your friends are ordering burgers and fries, it's almost impossible to forego eating. You don't have to starve, just eat some protein and you'll be fine. Scrambled eggs with no bread or potatoes, chicken breast without the wrap or a bowl of cottage cheese are all foods that can be found at any after-hours spot and you don't have to cry about the way you ate the next day. The other trick is to have quick proteins to grab from your fridge if you already came home. I'm one of those people who can't sleep when I'm starving. If I have a choice of eating something before bed or having insomnia, there is no debate. A few turkey slices, two hard boiled eggs, or some cheese and almonds don't break the caloric bank and should put you out like a light.

CHAPTER 8

VEGETARIAN DOESN'T = SKINNY

A lot of women tend to think that if they adopt a vegetarian lifestyle, they will automatically lose weight. Not so fast! You have to do it right in order to be healthy. There are a large percentage of vegetarians that eat way too many starchy carbohydrates in an attempt to cut out other foods. Just because you are eliminating meat, however, does not mean that there are no consequences to eating unlimited amounts of nuts, seeds, avocados, and other healthy oils. All the foods mentioned above are extremely healthy and necessary for vegetarians, but these are not "free foods" just because they come from the plant kingdom. I know firsthand from being a vegetarian for ten years.

When I was growing up, I lived with my aunt and uncle. My uncle ran a deli in Brooklyn and always came home with cold cuts like turkey, pastrami, corned beef, roast beef and basically any kind of processed fatty meat you can imagine. He was a big guy and every time I would sit down to eat a meal and watch my overweight extended family put that stuff in their mouths, it would make my stomach turn. I swore off meat for years but didn't know how to do vegetarian properly. Since I was athletic and knew that carbohydrates provided energy, I lived on plain pasta, dry bagels, cereal with skim milk, and frozen yogurt. No fat, no oil, no meat. I wasn't providing myself with enough nutrition and as a result my hair started thinning, my periods stopped and I gained weight.

A couple years later when I studied healing arts and yoga, I became more educated on the different vegetarian food options. I was more savvy to juicing and eating lots of organic fruits and vegetables. Nuts were my go-to snack or I'd put some almond butter on rice cakes. I lived on soy burgers, fake meats, and other foods that I believed were superior as meat substitutions. What I didn't know was that they also contained MSG, gluten, and - even worse - excitotoxins that can cause a host of health problems as well as accelerate aging. Tofu and tempeh are the exceptions since they are naturally fermented. While these hipster vegan restaurants that I would often eat at were still healthier than a fast food joint, my dishes were a far cry from healthy.

Macrobiotic restaurants also served my favorite dish called the Planet Platter — a combination of brown rice, seaweed, tofu and beans. I would eat a huge bowl and not think twice because all the ingredients were natural. In addition, I'd often top it off with a healthy cookie and a cup of vanilla soymilk. As I increased the fat in my diet, my periods seemed to regulate, yet I couldn't lose any weight. I thought it was because yoga was my only exercise and didn't do enough cardio.

It wasn't until I got into a serious relationship with a sports-watching "meat and potatoes" guy that I started to change my ways. He was in unbelievable shape and would often order a burger, grilled chicken or fish at every meal. When we would go out to eat I'd always piss him off because I'd just have vegetables and a potato or some rice. Since he wouldn't compromise and come with me to a vegetarian place, we'd eat in restaurants that didn't have any soy protein on the menu. I'd be starving from not having my beans or faux meat then end up overeating whatever starch was served...and still be unsatisfied. So I would go home and snack again while he was good for the night. He'd tease me and say that's why I couldn't lose weight because I was always eating. He said, "Why don't you just eat normal? An egg for breakfast or a piece of grilled fish or chicken every now and then won't kill you."

To keep the peace, I just shut up and took his advice. As committed as I was to my way of doing things, the results I was hoping for after many years had not manifested. I swapped out my almond butter and rice bread sandwiches in the morning for omelets or Greek yogurt. My lunches changed from veggie burgers and brown rice to grilled chicken salads. The dinners we'd have together were no longer my usual green salad and a potato but transitioned to fish with salad and vegetables. It wasn't like I was on a carbless diet. I still added starch to my meals such as a little quinoa, brown rice or sweet potato but it was a quarter of the amount I was eating previously. I was overeating those foods before because the lack of protein made me feel hungry. Even though plant proteins or nut butters may be equivalent in protein grams to a fleshy protein (i.e., meat, fish, poultry, or eggs), they are still incomplete proteins and don't keep you as full. That's why you may find yourself overeating grains. I realized I never actually felt well as a vegetarian until I started eating better quality proteins (which made me feel so much energetic and snack less). We're not talking about the nitrate-filled meats like hot dogs, bacon or lunch meats.

As I began to adopt my new lifestyle (which I wouldn't refer to as carnivorous since it was mostly fish and poultry), the pounds melted right off. My muscles that were defined from all the yoga postures were hidden under the extra weight I was holding until then. My biggest regret was that I waited so long being resistant to making those changes.

◆ ◆ ◆

Laurie, a new 21 year old model in New York City, was sent to me by her booker at the agency. She had a striking face yet every time she was sent on castings the clients would love her but tell her to come back after she lost a few pounds. Laurie by no means was a heavy girl, but her career would be short-lived if she didn't fit the designers' clothes. Being that she was originally a country girl, she had grown up on lots of comfort foods like fried chicken, chicken pot pie, beef chili, pork chops, bacon and eggs – basically things that cosmopolitan women would run from.

I knew working with her would be challenging because she had little education on nutrition; she only knew that the processed meats and fried foods she grew up on would sabotage her goals and the agency would drop her. She decided that the only way to slim down was to become a vegetarian and not eat the obvious junk foods like cakes and cookies and try to replace meat with soy alternatives. Here is a sample day of Laurie's diet when she came to me:

8 a.m.: One large bowl of cereal with rice milk and fresh fruit juice smoothie
10 a.m.: One handful of trail mix
12 p.m.: Two vegetarian sushi rolls and a banana from the gourmet deli on the way to castings
4 p.m.: One raisin oat bran muffin (also from a local deli) with soy chai latte
7 p.m.: Soy protein (Mock chicken or NOT Dogs) with baked potato, quinoa, or veggie dumplings
9 p.m.: Tofu ice cream sandwich or carob rice cakes for dessert

Laurie was not eating any real junk food, fatty meats or anything fried. Yet, her carbohydrate content and sugar intake was rather high. Check out how much she underestimated.

Her morning breakfast cereal was 170 calories and 35 grams of carbohydrates per serving. Although - if you looked closer – a serving was ½ cup. She was eating a full bowl which was about 3 servings and a half cup of rice milk – which is a very sugary and caloric beverage. The combined calories in her cereal bowl alone was about 560 calories 115 grams of carbohydrates and another 300 calories, 60 grams of carbohydrates and 30 grams of sugar in her smoothie. So essentially she was taking in almost 900 calories and roughly 175 grams of carbohydrates in just her breakfast.

That type of breakfast isn't particularly satisfying since it's so low in protein and high in refined carbohydrates (which lead to increased hunger). As her blood sugar spiked from this meal, in just a few hours it also plummeted, needing another fix.

Let's take a look at her morning snack choice which was trail mix. Depending on how big your handfuls are, they can set you back 500 calories. Trail mix also contains dried fruit which is several times more caloric than fresh fruit alone. While eating dried fruit and nuts sound good, not all brands are healthy. Many dried fruits contain sulphur dioxide as a preservative and the nuts are salted or soaked in hydrogenated oils which don't have the benefits of eating raw nuts. Even if you buy a health store brand, this kind of snack is not recommended unless you have the discipline to eat only a tablespoon!

Lunch time was difficult to find much to eat because she was running on casting calls. If you have visited NYC, you will quickly know that there is at least a deli or Starbucks™ on every other block for food emergencies. The deli is where she would get her vegetarian sushi rolls which are essentially rice filled with cucumber, avocado and sweet potato totaling close to 500 calories for 12 sushi pieces and a whopping 70 grams of carbohydrates. She would tax on a banana since she was still not quite full without the protein found within the fish of a normal sushi roll. A large banana is around 120 calories, 30 grams of carbohydrates and roughly 20 grams of sugar (although natural sugar). There are 620 calories in this lunch which is not terrible and relatively low-fat, but the carbohydrate content is very high (100 grams) yet again - like her breakfast - was raising her blood sugar levels.

By late afternoon Laurie would feel like she was crashing. Thankfully Starbucks™ was only a few steps from wherever she was on any particular day. A big high-fiber muffin and a soy chai latte would do the trick. Without even realizing it, she was consuming another 400 calories and 50 or 60 grams of carbohydrates with 20 grams of fat from the bran muffin alone; with the chai tea, she was adding another 200 calories and 40 grams of carbohydrates. The grand total of her snacking was 600 calories, close to 100 grams of carbohydrates along with a hefty dose of sugar and fat.

As dinnertime approached, she got to have her predictable soy-based meals since she was either cooking at home or ordering from her funky neighborhood health cafes in the trendy part of Brooklyn. Barbequed seitan, soy chicken nuggets, and tofu tempura were some of her favorites with a side of quinoa, rice or potato and usually sauce. "But these proteins are non-GMO," she argued "and must be healthy since they were prepared at a vegan restaurant or from a health food store." Her average dinner was another high-calorie, high fat and high carbohydrate meal that was setting her up for diet failure. A simply grilled piece of fish, poultry or meat would have been much healthier rather than trying to replicate it with a soy version that was masked in sauces to make it taste like the real thing.

Lastly, she had a sweet tooth and needed a little something before bed. Rice or soy-based ice creams would hit the spot, alternating with carob rice cakes which again were all snacks bought at a health food store. Portions were never monitored because it didn't actually seem like cheating with fake ice cream or fake chocolate. Laurie racked in another 200-300 calories, 40-50 grams of carbohydrates and 20 grams of fat that were eaten too late to be burned off. A few bites of gelato or some dark chocolate would have been the better choice since it's the real thing and you don't need as much to feel satisfied.

When we broke down her nutrition in our first session, she was mortified and couldn't believe how all her healthy vegetarian choices added up in calories, sugar, carbohydrates and fat. I explained that no matter how badly she wanted to succeed as a model, she would not get into her ideal shape by continuing what she was doing. Laurie could not see herself ever eating any kind of meat or poultry, but she was open to having eggs, dairy and an occasional piece of fish (organic options made her feel better about the quality, health benefits and treatment of the animals). I limited her soy foods to tofu and tempeh that were not marinated in sauces. She cut back significantly on her grains since the new proteins on her diet were more substantial and filled her up with half the amount of food. As a result, she slimmed down so much that she can now have one cheat day per week while having wiggle-room to fluctuate five pounds and still fit the designer clothes perfectly.

Whether you choose to be a vegetarian or not is a personal preference. In its original form – eating mostly fruits and vegetables, naturally fermented tofu, tempeh and small portions of beans, lentils, seeds, nuts and non glutenous grains – it's honestly more humane and better for the planet. If I wasn't so hungry all the time following that kind of program, I'd definitely do it myself. But if you are trying to replicate the modern American diet with a soy version and not watching your carbs (since you need to compensate for the lack of protein), you may want to rethink your strategy.

CHAPTER 9

GLUTEN-FREE MISTAKES YOU DON'T WANT TO MAKE

If you are from my generation, you will definitely remember the movie *Mean Girls* with Lindsay Lohan who played Cady, the new girl at school. The plot revolves around the clique of stuck-up popular girls called "The Plastics" whose leader Regina, was played by Rachel McAdams. Since Regina always behaved like an obnoxious bitch, Cady came up with a plan to get back at Regina by telling her about these special Swedish protein bars for weight loss called Kalteen Bars. The joke was that these bars actually made her gain weight but she had no idea what was in them since the labels were not in English. Kalteen Bars were what I call the former snacks I once lived on; they were wholesome, delicious and, yes, "gluten-free." I got them from the health food store and would often skip meals, relying on these dense, muffin/granola looking bars to fill me up instead. My rationale for eating them – including the fact they were "natural" and low-fat - was that I was having one less meal. So why did I pile on the pounds?

Roughly 18 years ago when I became a strict vegan and didn't touch sugar, there was no Whole Foods Market or easy accessibility to vegetarian salad bars that are now offered on every corner in Manhattan. When I was running on the go, I'd have to think in advance where there would be a health food store so I could grab something – somewhat reasonable –

in my mind. Rather than have an actual meal, my only option I thought was healthy were these giant, wheat-free, gluten-free, dairy-free cookies or rolled oat bars (Kalteen Bars) along with some kind of naturally sweetened tea, juice, or nut milk. I was doing physical labor from early in the morning until the evening with my clients and that was all following my 90-minute intensive 6 a.m. Ashtanga Yoga practice. Who actually gains weight with that kind of schedule on a vegan diet? I realized my biggest disaster was the "natural" cookies and oat snacks!

Here lies the problem with gluten-free snack foods. You trust what's in them because the package looks healthy and it appears to come from a credible source. I can assure you, though, that there is no stringent labeling regulation for these start-up health companies. Unless it's Kraft™ or Nabisco™ that has to watch out for a serious lawsuit, you better believe most are fudging the nutritional labels. Do yourself a favor and stay away! These seemingly healthy snacks may look small and harmless. You may even check the nutritional facts and it doesn't seem too bad. Then a few months later don't be surprised to see the label that once said "one serving per package 180 calories and 29 grams of carbohydrates" has now been changed to "200 calories and 33 grams of carbohydrates." And guess what? Now the label says each package is two servings. Accordingly, you are eating a 400 calorie snack, 66 grams of carbohydrates and throw in who knows how many grams of "natural sugar." Many small manufacturers will try to get away with as much as they can until they get busted.

If you are the kind of girl that skips a real lunch but instead grabs a dense, gluten-free chewy concoction that's the size of a baseball - watch out! Gluten-free cookies, muffins, pretzels, and oat bars will make you fat. Doesn't matter if they are 100% natural, organic, sweetened with honey or agave. At the end of the day, they are still snack foods that should be eaten recreationally. Don't let the tree hugger labels or the fact that they are sold at the health food store fool you.

Gluten-Free has become the new Fat-Free. Yet following the fat-free trend that was the hype in the 90's didn't prevent people from getting fatter. Agreed that a cookie with 25 grams of fat is still worse than a cookie with no fat, but a cookie is still a cookie. Eating a gluten-free bowl of pasta or macaroni and cheese for dinner will still make you gain weight unless you plan to use those carbs to go run a marathon.

Let me preface my opinion by also stating that I happen to follow a gluten-free diet. I also ask that most of my clients go gluten-free as well regardless if they suffer or not from Celiac Disease. From a health perspective, I see improvements across the board when gluten is eliminated from the diet. Giadin, a protein found in gluten, tends to cause inflammation in many people. Inflammation also causes weight gain. Gluten intolerance may additionally reveal itself through digestive problems, achy joints, auto-immune disease, skin conditions, headaches and possibly more for people who are sensitive. So yes I feel avoiding foods with gluten is good. It's less complicated to just consume foods that are naturally gluten-free such as fruits, vegetables, fish and poultry along with red meat, beans, legumes, soy products and grains in limited quantities. Don't be tempted by foods that are substituted with gluten-free flours or starches to make an otherwise gluten-containing product now be considered healthy.

For example, if you eat gluten-free pasta, the wheat and gluten have been removed but now it's substituted with rice, potato starch or corn. The same goes for gluten-free bread, cereals etc. What makes this worse is that the gluten-free replications almost always contain more carbohydrates and calories. Do yourself a favor and check out a box of whole wheat bread versus gluten-free rice bread. Many times one slice is double the calories and carbs. I'm not a fan of either, but you should know what you're getting into. "Gluten-free pizza" is not a smart substitution when trying to lose weight. Additionally, gluten-free products typically have less fiber and are higher on the glycemic index. This will raise your blood sugar more quickly, fill you up less, and have you craving more food once you've finished. If your kitchen cabinets have a surplus of gluten-free goodies, you don't need throw everything out. Simply see it as a treat or use the remains for a dinner party and don't restock. Some swaps that I recommend for your favorite man-made, gluten-free foods are the following.

Gluten-free pasta Shirataki noodles. These are made from tofu and an entire bag is only 6 grams of carbohydrates and 40 calories. It's not exactly the same as having a bowl of pasta, but if you dress it up with some meatballs, salmon or grilled chicken with some fresh tomato sauce or olive oil and garlic with a side of broccoli, you now have a tasty meal that you didn't blow a workout for.

Sandwich Bread Udi's™ makes a decent gluten-free bread if you have an occasional sandwich. Yet, if your preference is to have sandwiches all the time, try stuffing your protein such as tuna, turkey, or burgers in cabbage leaves, Portobello mushroom or a large bell pepper. To fatten it up, add on lettuce, avocado, and alfalfa sprouts. If that doesn't fill you up, have a side of roasted yellow, green, butternut squash or beets instead of chips or French fries.

Desserts (cookies, cakes, and pastries) We already went over that gluten-free snacks are not the best swaps. Instead have two squares of 80% organic dark chocolate with a few raw almonds or a baked apple or pear with cinnamon. You can also sprinkle a few crumbs of gluten-free granola and add stevia before baking and it makes it taste like you are eating pie. Yet it's perfectly portioned without the guilt…

It may sound like I'm advocating a very low-carb diet. But the case for most people is we end up making up the carbohydrates regardless if we want to live a normal existence. If you go to a friend's house for a meal or out to dinner, it's okay to let yourself go a little. So by being conscious on your own time, you have the room to be less strict in public as long as you're open about being gluten-free. It's totally accepted now that no one will think it's strange. Yet, if you're in a summer share house with friends and start making sandwiches wrapped in cucumber slices they will think you're a nut job! So know your company and make choices to the best of your ability with the foods that are being served. Don't piss off your boyfriend's mom by not eating a thing at their place upstate over the weekend. Go with the flow, knowing you will go back to your routine in the comfort of your own kitchen.

Alternatively, if you go to a restaurant with a gluten-free menu, it's better to bypass the gluten-free pastas or breads for the novelty. Instead, choose from carbohydrates that are higher in fiber and naturally gluten-free. Quinoa, sweet potato, brown rice, and butternut squash make the best side dishes. But remember, it's not in unlimited quantities. These starchy foods are best if eaten earlier in the day rather than at night.

To live the Gluten-Free lifestyle, here are my takeaways to get the most benefit.

#1. Ask yourself, "Was this product manufactured to be gluten-free? Or is this a naturally gluten-free food?"

#2. Follow as many of my suggested food swaps that are realistic when you are in the privacy of your own home (so people don't laugh and discourage you) and go easy on the grains (even if gluten-free). Eat double portions of green leafy and starchy vegetables for extra fiber and fullness.

#3. Aside from high-quality protein bars and shakes (which we will discuss later in another chapter) abandon the habit of eating gluten-free snack foods. This means anything that comes in a box, bag, or contains a wrapper. You can eat them recreationally – but understand it's not much better for your figure than eating a brownie or slice of cheesecake.

CHAPTER 10

THE DARK SIDE OF JUICING

It's 2015 and this is a typical scene as the girls walk out of their Bikram Yoga studio, ©Barry's Bootcamp or Soul Cycle™. Everyone is sporting the high-tech athletic wear and hoping the workout will improve the way they look in it. Now to prepare for - or finish off - their class, they go for a large green juice which has replaced the days of a sugar-free, no whip, non-fat vanilla latte.

So long to just drinking plain old lemon water in a thermos for detoxification. Juicing has become so fashionable that if you haven't partaken in a juice cleanse within the past six months you might even start to be feeling lame. For many, it wouldn't be sufficient to just grind up some vegetables and pour them in a cup to go. Juice culture has taken over cities by storm and people are loyal to only drinking the best brands. Why else would a twenty-something PR executive that barely makes $50k a year (with two roommates struggling to get by) spend $12 on a cup of fancy kale?

Don't think I'm knocking the concept of juicing all together. I was an avid juicer back in the late 90's during my vegan era and living in Alphabet City- the East Village of Manhattan. Most of the people in my neighborhood were either tattooed vegetarian hipsters or artists with a few heroin addicts sprinkled in on every corner. Probably not much different than the streets of Haight Ashbury in San Francisco. I think they liked the proximity to Thompson Square Park which was notorious for being a haven of

The Dark Side of Juicing

anything that could be injected through a needle. They have since cleaned up the neighborhood and populated it with rich NYU kids and studio apartments going for $3000 a month. I guess the junkies had to find a new home somewhere in Brooklyn or Queens.

Health food stores, vegan restaurants, vintage boutiques, indie movie theaters and rock and roll joints were what gave the neighborhood its flavor. If you went to a yoga class, ate a veggie burger or had a spinach and carrot juice for lunch, you didn't brag about it. That was just what was expected as part of an everyday normal existence. Mornings after yoga I'd share the rush hour subway with all the yuppies headed to Wall Street. I'd be in my sweaty, non-fashionable spandex drinking something green, while they were reading The NY Times with a coffee in hand and wearing suits. They probably thought I was some tree-hugging weirdo. Remember, these were the days before the sexy Lulu Lemon™ couture and juice franchises began popping up everywhere.

Sometimes I'd take on juicing for three days up to a full week. It was totally miserable. I would be dizzy for days from overdosing on natural sugar and have to train my mind to not pay attention to the hunger. After the cleanse I maybe lost a pound or possibly two but nothing of value in terms of health benefit. If you eat a crappy diet of processed and artificial foods, you may see a shift with juicing because you are eliminating bad food and alcohol (for the time being) and, therefore, cutting back on calories but not necessarily because juices are amazing. My diet was already rich in fruits and vegetables and I felt a hundred times better eating those foods rather than drinking them. Yes, juicing is rich in nutrients – but once the pulp and fiber are removed, the sugar from the juice enters the bloodstream much more quickly than if you were eating an actual fruit or vegetable in its whole form. The other issue with juicing as a meal replacement is that there is not sufficient protein. When you take fiber and protein out of the equation, hunger is usually inevitable.

If you are familiar with the principals of Yin and Yang, you will understand that food is categorized in many cultures by being more of one than the other. Practicing Chinese Medicine, Taoisim, and following a macrobiotic diet combines foods that have both Yin and Yang properties to maintain nutritional balance. Yin foods such as raw fruit, vegetables, juices, and sugars are cooling, while Yang foods such as cooked root vegetables, eggs, meat, and spices are warming. In the wintertime you don't want to do a week-long juice cleanse which is not only cooling to the body but also creates the perfect damp environment for candida, (possible yeast infection), water retention and, yes, depression too. Yang foods in excess aren't good, either, since they can be too heating and create too much fiery energy. Ideally, your diet should contain a little of both. If you are obsessed with having 10 servings of vegetables a day, cook or stir-fry your vegetables with garlic or ginger to keep the right constitution of Yin and Yang. It's not advised to drink down multiple stalks of raw spinach and chlorella powder.

To reap the benefits of juicing, you will probably be more successful doing it in small doses such as one day a week in spring or summer. Otherwise, long-term juicing can just be depleting. I don't believe juicing is inherently bad and I'm all for giving the digestive system a break. I incorporate juices every so often into my diet for the convenience of getting greens on the go when there is no time to sit down for a salad. When I'm running to appointments and it's either starve or have something quick on the subway that's not messy, I'll often pick up two pre-peeled hard-boiled eggs with an organic green juice. My issue with juicing is that many people make the transition from eating a diet that's not thoughtful (fried foods, processed meats, cheeses, pastries, sodas, alcohol, etc.) and then jump ship to a juice cleanse the next day as an attempt to quickly clean up their diet and lose weight in the process.

Juice cleanses should be eased into by slowly improving the diet at least a week before going cold turkey on bad food. Cutting out inflammatory foods such as wheat, sugar, red meat, dirty beverages, etc. and sticking to easy to digest proteins, fruits and vegetables are the only safe way to make the transition. You don't want to have a bipolar attitude about de-toxing and re-toxing. I'm talking about swinging from crappy foods, becoming a purist for five days, and then going back to your old ways. This will only slow your metabolism and none of the benefits will stick if juicing is viewed as a "get out of jail free" card after misbehaving.

If you drink juices as a daily snack for the health benefits in addition to your regular diet, there are still downsides. If your greens contain some apple, one or two whole apples may be used for that hint of apple flavor. Carrot juice often uses four sticks for one serving. The same applies to quantities of beets, oranges, bananas, berries or whatever else gives your drink its sweetness. This really adds up in terms of sugar and calories and even contain more than many meals. You would be more satisfied eating these foods whole since the fiber is left intact, unlike the end result after liquefying these fruits and vegetables. Even when juicing leafy greens, a whole bushel of kale, spinach, broccoli or cabbage may be used for a 12 ounce serving. While that sounds like the healthiest thing ever, this is not the case if you have an underactive thyroid. Hypothyroidism (low thyroid function) can be a huge contributor to weight gain. These cruciferous vegetables in their raw form can further suppress thyroid function and actually make you heavier.

The path of juicing does not ultimately lead to weight loss. Yet, short term intermittent fasting (12-24 hours) done as a ritual before prayer or meditation with lemon water or juice is usually safe and can enhance your practice. But before you break the bank on your Green habit, the money would be better spent on buying organic whole foods, fruits and vegetables.

CHAPTER 11

SNACKS THAT CAN SABOTAGE OR KEEP YOU SKINNY

If you're physically active or have long stretches of time in between meals, snacking doesn't have to be a diet saboteur. The problem is girls who diet usually snack on the wrong things. Many of the fashion models that I work with to stay in shape enthusiastically tell me how they pack healthy snacks to run around with on casting calls. "So what's usually in your bag?" I ask. The more impressive responses are often carrot sticks, dried seaweed, kale chips, or organic blueberries. These are all good things but to have any sense of satiety you need to eat the entire bag or box (which is typically more than one serving size). None of these snacks are that high in calories, yet if you look at the carbohydrate or sugar content, it's up there. Not to mention the protein is almost nil. So after having your treat, chances are you will still be craving something else. There is no fullness factor and it gives you no protection against being ravenous when meal time rolls around again.

The other responses I get regarding snacks are especially problematic for spiking insulin levels and weight gain. These include popcorn, rice cakes, granola bars, crackers and pretzels (even the organic/non-gmo kind). If you thought the carbohydrate content was high in the earlier snacks I mentioned, these "healthy marketed" options are even worse and relatively low in nutrient value. Deficient in protein, these snack foods are quickly digested, converted into sugar and subsequently stored as fat. High carb snacks lacking protein often take hefty portions to be filling. So it's easy to eat 2-3 servings in a blink while being totally unaware that this is calorically equivalent to a meal.

I happen to be a fan of nuts and seeds. Almonds, cashews, walnuts, pistachios, chia seeds, flax seeds etc. all have a home in my pantry, but you need to know if you can stick to portions. For many girls, these snacks are off limits. Going to the health food store and scooping out these snacks by the pound from one of those bins into a plastic baggy can be trouble. It's very easy to just eat right out of the bag without first portioning your servings. You can literally blow through hundreds to thousands of calories! Yes, these snacks all contain "good fat." In large quantities, however, you are setting yourself up for weight gain. A handful of nuts or seeds is roughly considered a serving and equivalent to one ounce; just be sure you can stop right there. Be aware that all nuts don't calorically come out to be the same. Keep these nutritional facts in mind.

- Almonds are one of the least caloric nuts for their serving size. For a portion of 23, they contain 160 calories, 14 grams of fat and 6 grams of protein.
- Cashews are 17 nuts per serving for the same 160 calories and 14 grams of fat with about 5 grams of protein.
- Walnuts are a little more fattening with 14 halves as a serving equaling 190 calories, 18 grams of fat and 4 grams of protein.
- Pistachios, (although a little annoying to eat without a garbage can nearby) are the best calorically in terms of serving size. You get 46 nuts for 160 calories, 13 grams of fat and 6 grams of protein.

If you enjoy peanuts, they are technically not nuts; they are legumes. While they have some redeeming qualities such as healthy monounsaturated fats, fiber and nutrients good for preventing heart disease down the road, they are frequently contaminated with a carcinogenic mold called aflatoxin. From a weight loss perspective, they are highly caloric, not as nutritious as the other nuts mentioned and are very difficult to portion out.

So what about peanut butter and almond butter? Almond butter over peanut butter wins, although it really depends what you put your almond butter on during snack time. Almond butter on rice cakes can be a diet disaster. For 2 rice cakes and 1 tbsp of almond butter on each cake, you will rack in over 300 calories and 20 grams of fat. I also know girls who like to stick a spoon in the peanut butter or almond butter and eat several bites (considering that their protein intake for the day). Five hundred calories and 50 grams of fat later, they wonder why they are not losing weight! A serving is just one tbsp. If you are disciplined enough to do that and make your spoonful last on a few celery sticks or an apple, then go for it.

Chia seeds, flax seeds, or any kind of "Super Seed" can be a good source of fiber in a shake or a topping on your salad, but not something you want to snack on by the handfuls. At roughly 70 calories per tbsp, they make better pairings with other meals rather than a stand-alone snack.

Protein powders can be a very smart snack but need to be chosen wisely. I like to carry a small shaker bottle with me to work with a single serving of protein powder. When my blood sugar gets low, I just add a little water and voila! I have a shake with no blender required. My rules about protein powders are that they should be under 200 calories, over 10 grams of protein and under 30 grams of carbohydrates. For caloric reasons, they should only be mixed with water and not milk, milk substitutes, or coconut water. Additionally, if you want to add a tbsp of seeds, a handful of berries, and/or some raw cacao, you need to calculate that extra pairing and make sure not to exceed the 200 calorie mark. Once you start making a "Super Shake" all tricked out with a million ingredients, it's no longer a snack — it's a meal!

Energy bars - if chosen correctly - can save you on the go, but if you buy the wrong kind you may be eating something no better than a glorified candy bar. Just like protein shakes, I don't want my female clients eating bars that are over 200 calories, over 30 grams of carbohydrates and contain more than 10 grams of fat. Additionally, make sure it contains at least 10 grams of protein. Many bars on the market are touted as healthy and natural because they are rich in nuts, seeds and fruit. A bar like this usually can run between 200-300 calories with 10-15 grams of fat and under 6 grams of protein. It's a little deceptive because we associate nuts and seeds to be high-protein ingredients. After eating one of these bars, I promise you will still be hungry since it lacks protein and now you just wasted a few hundred calories. The higher protein, high-fiber bars will help to balance your blood sugar, keep you fuller longer and help you to eat less at your next meal. Just be careful to not have more than one bar a day since they can be addictive!

My other snacks of choice are:

- **Edamame** You can boil this at home and pack in a ziplock bag if on the go. It tastes good either hot or cold. One serving is around 180 calories with 17 grams of protein and 8 grams of fiber.
- **Hard Boiled Eggs** You can make them yourself or pick them up at most delis or convenience stores. One egg is around 70 calories and 6 grams of protein.
- **Greek Yogurt** The low-fat plain kind is around 150 calories and 20 grams of protein in a single serving.
- **String Cheese** An unprocessed, organic string cheese can be found at any health food store and is about 80 calories per serving and 6 grams of protein.

Rather than worry about the implications of snacking, the truth is that it can actually save you. I've never walked into a Thanksgiving meal or holiday dinner feeling too hungry. Having a small portion of something healthy in your body will always prevent overeating. It makes you not need to order an appetizer at dinner or nibble on bread rolls before your meal arrives. As a rule, I always have a high protein snack two hours prior to going out for a meal. That's the biggest insurance for not regretfully overdoing it – especially at dinner time. We can try to count on self-control but it's not reliable when you're starving. At the end of the day we're all like animals at feeding time. Without having a snack to reduce those instinctive urges to eat everything in front of us, we're likely to consume way more than we bargained for. So that 200 calories you may have been afraid to invest in at snack time has now turned into an additional 1000 calories. Between the starters, bread and now finishing your entire entrée, you just blew your diet - whereas a less hungry girl would have only eaten half the amount.

CHAPTER 12

WHAT'S LURKING IN YOUR SAUCES, DRESSINGS AND CONDIMENTS?

On any given night after work, it's always a zoo at a local health food chain salad bar (that shall remain nameless). As the patrons grab their eco-friendly paper boxes and begin filling them with salad stuffings, they barely glance over the ingredients that are transparently on display in front of their faces. That's because there is trust that this health food giant would only serve foods that are good for overall health and wellness. What you need to know, however, is that most people working in the kitchen are not even educated on nutrition. The health food restaurant business is not always run very different from a McDonalds™ or Subway™ except more exotic foods are being including in the daily selections. It also does not mean that everything served is organic, wild, or grass fed. Many cooks are pressured to prep food quickly, make it taste good and assure their bosses that everything is flowing smoothly. It's not that they don't care about your health, but the ingredients in those fancy dishes and salad bars are usually frightening.

The first time I ever examined the salad bar ingredients at my favorite health café, I was mortified. Why did heavy cream and wheat need to be added to my tomato soup? Were the tomatoes organic and if not, could they have been GMO? Then I moved on to the tuna and didn't understand why there was soy sauce, eggs and sugar in some tuna that would have been easily delicious just plain. I kept walking and stopped at the cod that smelled so good. Then I realized it had butter as one of the main ingredients along with orange juice and some other odd pairings to give it flavor. I figured I'd just keep it simple and have tofu as a last resort until I noticed the sign said "contains wheat". Huh? I'm gluten-free and can't have wheat. This is not an ingredient in naturally fermented tofu.

The experience of trying to settle on a meal became even more disconcerting as I perused every single dish - including the vegetables. I didn't want my Brussels sprouts to be soaked in sugary organic maple syrup with salty bacon bits. No wonder why years of eating at health food cafés would give me stomachaches. I had always believed that the food was clean because it came from a vendor I trusted. How could they not be more selective with their recipes?

Here lies the dilemma in eating prepared foods. Even the foods we make at home often become tainted when we start adding marinades, sauces or salad dressings. Did you ever really look at the amount of sugar and corn syrup in a bottle of ketchup or honey Dijon mustard? How many of us actually take the time to dissect the ingredients? Especially if those condiments are marketed as healthy products, it becomes more confusing. Many times the mainstream unhealthy ingredients are replaced with sneaky ingredients to make it taste better and we don't understand how to decode the labels. For example, people who are sensitive to Monosodium Glutamate (MSG) may look for those words specifically. Yet it can be disguised as glutamic acid, hydrolyzed protein, autolyzed yeast or bouillon. MSG can cause migraines, fatigue, diarrhea, or even difficulty breathing. Another hidden ingredient that comes from seaweed called Carrageenan is often found in nut milks, creams, and salad dressing. Carrageenan sounds healthy since there is a mental association between seaweed, the ocean, and anything natural and yet it can trigger an allergic response and wreak havoc on the digestive system. Anyone that suffers from sensitive bowels can have a flare up right after eating anything formulated with it. Clients will often come to me and complain about digestive troubles or not losing weight while following a low-carb, low-fat, mostly grain-free diet. My first question is usually, "Where do you get your meals from?" I hear answers such as, "I go to the same place every day and get the lemon chicken with broccoli or the spiced tofu soup from the Vietnamese place." They have no idea how much sodium, sugar, fat or calories are laced in each dish.

Have you ever stopped to think what's inside sushi? Most people think it's just simple fish, seaweed and rice. Many times, though, it has added teriyaki sauce, eel sauce, spicy sauce, mayonnaise etc. which all contain wheat (unacceptable on a gluten-free diet), sugar and crazy amounts of sodium. Most people don't eat the sushi without soy sauce, either. Even the low-sodium version is a joke which racks in about 500mg of sodium per tablespoon. Do you know anyone who actually portions out their soy sauce with a spoon to not go overboard?

While sushi is not a low calorie food, it's still not the worst thing calorically. The issue with ethnic foods is their sauces. Whether you eat a dish from Japan, China, India, Italy, or American style barbeque, you are at risk from what your meals are bathing in. Have you ever watched one of those cooking competitions on television? First the chef may add a large dollop of butter, then some barbeque sauce, add on a few sprinkles of sugar, a heap of salt, a cup of wine and possibly even a schmear of lard "pig fat" (sorry kosher girls – always ask your waiter). Once you wrap your head around that, I don't think you need me to tell you what all those ingredients will do to your figure.

One of the best habits you can take on is to buy your food raw and plain at the salad bar and in a restaurant ask for sauce on the side. Personally I would try to do all together without the sauce and drizzle your own olive oil, lemon, salt and pepper on to your own dish. If you are not one to be fussy when dining out, you can still do it with class and humor. Let's role play.

You Excuse me waiter. I hate to be a pain in the ass, but I have several food allergies and need to be very careful with the way my food is prepared. Would you mind telling the very talented chef that although his cooking is delicious, I need to have my meal simply grilled with no sauce. Please send him my apologies and ask him kindly not to spit in my food. (Now smile at waiter, and then smile at your company).

Just be a lady, act like it's no big deal and carry on with your conversation. I do this all the time and understand on dates it can make you look a little prissy. As long as you act cool and don't judge him for his eating habits, you can probably get away with it. While guys love a girl who can get down with a cheese burger and fries, that unfairly seems to apply when she also has an incredible metabolism. Sorry guys, most of us can't eat like a truck driver and then fulfill your expectations when we're wearing lingerie.

When you are cooking at home, you should still be aware of what you prepare your meals with. The one exception is when you are expecting company. In that case, go ahead and complete your salad with a peppercorn dressing, marinate your meat overnight in barbeque glaze, or add a lemon butter reduction to your scallops and pasta. This is for special occasions but when you are cooking for one, toss the sauce.

Your skinny girl staples are olive oil, lemon, garlic, onion, ginger, sea salt, pepper, and as many crazy spices you can get creative with. Feel free to knock yourself out with chili peppers or curry powder if the idea of bland food seems like a punishment. Ditching the sauce doesn't have to be flavorless. You may have also noticed that I mentioned salt on that list. That's because if you are preparing a food from scratch and it's sauce-free, it won't have any sodium to begin with. A sprinkle of sea salt contains much less sodium then a well dressed salad (even if you haven't touched the salt shaker).

To satisfy a sweet tooth, honey and agave are often used as "natural" condiments. While they both have health benefits, minerals, antioxidants and even some healing properties, they are also high in calories, fructose and carbohydrates. One tablespoon of honey or agave actually contains more calories than a tablespoon of sugar. If you are diabetic, have blood sugar issues or trying to lose weight, these natural condiments are not a good idea. The next time you want to sweeten up your tea or Greek yogurt, opt for Stevia™ instead; this plant-based sweetener does not contain calories. If you're on a health kick, it's the best choice for giving into your cravings without the cancer-causing saccharin or aspartame.

CHAPTER 13

GOT CELLULITE?

Doesn't matter if you're thick or thin, cellulite does not discriminate. I know firsthand that no matter how skinny I am, the weight never seems to disappear from my ass. It's the only area of my body that is disproportionate to the rest of my otherwise small frame. In many ways I guess that's a good thing considering I have no boobs so the curvy bottom makes me feel more womanly. In pants or a fitted skirt it has the appearance of looking pretty firm, but truth be told it's jiggly. While I've been very athletic most of my life, I've had a dimply butt since I can remember hitting puberty.

There are many reasons why females develop cellulite and it's not necessarily because they are overweight or lack discipline. In fact, I had a conversation with Dr. Lionel Bissoon, a leading physician in Manhattan that treats this condition and was surprised to learn that cellulite is more prominent in thin women. According to him, thicker women have larger bone structures that seem to provide more "room for growth" if you will. Even as their fat cells grow larger, these women seem to "wear" the extra weight well. If you have a smaller build, the cellulite appears more obvious.

Dr. Bissoon explained that most people think cellulite develops as a result of either poor nutrition or lack of exercise. While a healthier lifestyle can reduce the appearance of cellulite, it's not always the reason it showed up in the first place. Yet, he was clear to communicate that a sedentary lifestyle and eating an unhealthy diet obviously won't improve the situation. There are mainstream foods we should steer clear of for a number of health reasons besides a mushy bottom. Foods that specifically can worsen cellulite formation are those that are processed and/or contain a lot of sugar, chemicals, and artificial sweeteners. In addition to offering little or no nutritional value, they can become toxic to the system. Having a toxic buildup can subsequently slow down circulation and reduce skin elasticity, thus making cellulite more visible.

The best nutritional habits to take on are to stay hydrated with purified water (fresh lemon optional) along with foods that work as natural diuretics. Organic vegetables such as asparagus, cucumbers, celery and leafy greens do exactly that and are helpful for de-toxing. You can also improve blood vessel health and circulation with high quality foods high in omega-3 and 6 fatty acids such as wild salmon, sardines, olive oil, raw nuts and avocados. There have been studies to suggest that Vitamin C can help to build collagen and reduce the appearance of cellulite. Vitamin C is also an antioxidant that is good for the skin and that's why it is used in so many topical skin care creams. Oranges, berries and pineapple are some of the best sources. They should be eaten whole rather than juiced because of the high sugar content. The extra calories of the juices will cause weight gain and cancel out any of the positive effects of their nutrients.

One key reason for cellulite formation, Dr. Bisson noted is declining estrogen levels as we age. Keep in mind that you don't have to be middle-aged to see your estrogen levels drop. It can happen as early as your 20's. He brought up a great point about "primitive" women living in rural countries. They tend to eat more organic foods than their U.S. counterparts; they consume larger quantities of plants and naturally occurring soy foods which contain phyto-estrogens. These plant estrogens mimic the effects of naturally occurring estrogens in the body. Accordingly, these women don't suffer many of the symptoms that we do here in American culture.

Dr. Bissoon also remarked that in addition to walking, working the fields, clearly living a less sedentary lifestyle, and not eating the highly refined and processed Standard American Diet, these primitive women don't wear restrictive clothing. Many don't even wear underwear. He went on to make the argument why keeping your bottom panty-free or in a thong is a great habit to get into. Wearing grandma underwear at a young age can be damaging in that it contains elastic that stretches across the buttocks and upper thighs, constricts the flow of blood and compresses the lymphatic vessels which all bring on the cellulite. Sometimes the cellulite dimples are even oriented to the contour of the panty lines. While women often believe tight underwear supports a tight butt, it ends up applying too much compression and works like a tourniquet that completely stops circulation.

Here are Dr. Bissoon's anti-cellulite rules for choosing your panties:

1. No elastic over the buttocks.
2. No elastic over the groin area.
3. Elastic is okay at the waist.
4. Use underwear with lace instead of elastic.
5. Preferable to wear thongs/G-strings.
6. Not wearing underwear is an option.
7. Stockings/pantyhose are beneficial.
8. Sleep in the nude or a pull-over nighty.
9. Don't wear underwear and pantyhose together.

Cellulite may also be due to genetics. If you are already predisposed to cellulite (as I was at a young age) the practice of being calorie conscious, eating mostly organic foods, and doing exercises such as walking, cycling, squats, lunges and yoga may help firm your butt and thighs. It's not a cure, however. Nor is it insurance if you take to wearing teeny tiny underwear. These can only be preventative measures to stop the problem from getting worse. Once cellulite arrives, it will most likely require additional outside support to really nip it in the bud. Even if you've become successful with a weight loss program, cellulite is one of those annoying things like stretch marks. It may stay with you eternally unless you are open to taking cosmetic measures. I've never known anyone to have real success with topical creams or potions, but there is hope without having to go under the knife. Non-surgical treatments that Dr. Bissoon has found to be most helpful are Mesotherapy and Subcision.

Mesotherapy, discovered in 1952 by French physician Dr. Michael Pistor, is the practice of delivering microinjections of conventional or homeopathic medications (and/or vitamins) under the skin to directly treat the areas where the condition exists. When treating cellulite, multiple injections are given in rows over the affected area. While the treatments may initially produce some bruising, it's only temporary and worth the eventual outcome.

Subcision is an outpatient procedure that targets the connective tissues under the skin, using a special hypodermic needle. It sounds scarier than it is but it's relatively pain-free. Subcision can be the most effective when performed in conjunction with Mesotherapy.

I'd also like to mention an anti-cellulite treatment called Vaser Shape. While the dimples on my butt never really bothered me enough to take action, I was curious if this treatment could actually iron them out. I went through a series of sessions at Park Avenue Aesthetics with Dr. Douglas Senderoff. Vaser Shape uses low frequency ultrasound energy to the fatty tissue layer below the surface of the skin. The treatment uses a very high heat and essentially felt like a really hot massage on my ass. After five visits, my butt literally went from bumpy to smooth. Almost three decades of sports and an extremely disciplined diet just couldn't produce those kinds of results.

One piece of advice from Dr. Bissoon – "Don't wait until the summer to do any of these procedures. They all require a number of visits and you want to give yourself time to heal before you make that beachfront appearance. Plan ahead and get moving on it during the winter when you can hide out with no pressure on timing."

Regardless of what method you pursue to conquer your cellulite once and for all, you can't get lazy or it will come back. Regressing to bad eating habits or lack of physical activity can trigger its return. And so can a big pair of panties.

CHAPTER 14

WEIGHT LOSS SLIP UPS: TIPS FROM A HOLLYWOOD TRAINER

It's completely frustrating to have a solid exercise routine, yet not see the fruits of your labor. I definitely observe a lot of familiar girls at the gym who I've noticed over the years on the same training schedule. They are diligent about working out all the time and are still noticeably chunky. Well, there are a couple of things they are missing. I decided to refer to Brett Hoebel, author of *The 20 Minute Body* and former trainer on *The Biggest Loser* to share some of his expert advice and to help identify where you may be going wrong.

Brett didn't always have the muscular body of an Adonis combined with his martial arts talents to maneuver like Bruce Lee. And yet, he makes it look so effortless. In fact, Brett with his smooth moves and perfect physique was once bullied for being a chubby kid. (There's hope for all of us)! That was actually the catalyst to propel him to change his ways, take his health seriously and become the inspiration that he is today.

Brett's Take on Women and Weight Lifting While it's not a common sight at most gyms, you've probably seen some very athletic women with big, bulky muscles. Naturally this had led many women to be wary of weights. The assumption is that any use of resistance training will cause a gain of pounds and inches or that it could compromise the look they are going for. Although Brett says it's possible to get bulky if you train the wrong way, it's very unlikely. Typically, this means increasingly heavy weights done with particular sets - and – reps schemes designed to build that kind of muscle. So it can happen. It's just not an easy thing for women to do, however, so don't let that scare you away from strength training.

According to Brett, the key to everything is muscle – you have to train it, gain it, and maintain it in order to keep everything metabolic. That does not mean you need to have the muscles of a bodybuilder to see results although this kind of training speeds up metabolism so you are burning fat and calories around the clock – yes, even at rest. While long, steady cardio generally burns a lot of calories during a workout, (running, hiking, biking, walking), to elevate metabolism and maintain muscle –you have to do both.

Mindset and Mantras Brett is a huge believer in the power of mantras to inspire results, whether it's in the gym, at work or in your personal life. Find a mantra each week that expresses the deepest idea about what you want to achieve, and repeat it – silently or aloud - as often as you can to reinforce that concept. It can be funny, serious, inspirational, or reflective. It's meant to be an expression of your own personality. Make sure it's fresh, has real energy and inspires you.

When you choose your mantra, write it down and post it where you're going to see it a lot. It could be a screensaver on your computer or phone, taped to a corkboard in your office, or posted on your bathroom mirror so that you see it first thing in the morning. These don't have to be Shakespearean, just simple and meaningful to you.

Your Diet Can Be Your Saboteur Brett says that exercise creates the stimulus for change, your mindset helps you stay consistent, but you need the right nutrition to really see the results you are looking for. This is also the part that trips up most people. "I've had clients over the years who train with me like a beast session after session but after a while we stop seeing results. When I notice stalls like this, I don't ask the clients to train harder or switch up their program. I ask them what they are eating. And 99 percent of the time, they're making mistakes in one or more key areas of their diet. Once we address those problems, the inches and pounds start coming off again." Brett cautions against white starch, preservatives, high-sugar, high-fat, and high-sodium foods which make it nearly impossible to burn fat, shed water and keep insulin levels in check for visible weight loss. Instead, he suggests going "lean, clean and green" which is essentially filling your diet with lean sources of protein, clean unprocessed foods, and lots of greens (and other brightly colored) vegetables.

Being that I'm a New Yorker and Brett lives in LA, there are also some common mistakes that people who like to party get in trouble with. He calls them the "Overdoers." These are ones who like to train hard by day and hit the town by night. Brett insists how recovering from workouts with adequate sleep is vital. The body actually changes during rest and recovery. Without sufficient rest, your body increases production of the stress hormone cortisol, which can actually eat away at muscle tissue and cause you to accumulate belly fat.

The other problem with living in a town that has a great night life is the temptation of drinking too much. He talks about how alcohol is the ultimate empty calorie. When people ask him for tips on how to lose weight, he tells them the number one thing to cut out is alcohol. That's because alcohol turns right into sugar when it hits your liver. And a "wine pour" at most restaurants is much larger than the recommended five ounces. It's like eating an extra meal at midnight and still expecting to lose weight. In other words, it's not going to happen.

Brett explains alcohol is also risky because our bodies naturally want to eat when we're drinking in order to absorb and metabolize the alcohol.

That can lead to more unwanted calories. The worst decisions typically happen when we drink. He jokes about who shows up sober at 2 a.m. for pancakes at IHOP? Brett doesn't say to give up alcohol completely, but asks you to be really honest about the amount you drink if you truly want to lose weight. Here are his tips for enjoying alcohol in a way that will minimize its impact on your body.

- Decide before you go out how much you're going to drink or if you're going to drink at all. If you are drinking to be social, set a strict limit. One drink for women and two drinks for men if you're seriously committed to weight loss.
- Don't drink too late in the evening or you won't sleep well because you'll be waking up in the middle of the night to go to the bathroom and because alcohol interrupts natural sleep cycles.
- Red wine is one of the better options because it contains compounds that promote heart health. A glass of red wine has generally less sugar than the standard four-ounce well drink and a four- ounce well drink is usually less sugary than sweet cocktails, which are packed with calories. A four ounce MaiTai – which is a blend of lime juice, curacao, light and dark rum - can contain 250 or more calories and 18 grams of sugar, while a five-ounce "pour" of red wine has about 125 calories and less than five grams of sugar.
- Lighter colored alcoholic drinks are "cleaner" (i.e., vodka with club soda), but it's still important to gulp water between drinks so that you don't get too tipsy and accidentally overindulge. Drinking water also keeps your stomach full, which will prevent the late-night drive-thru run or stumbling into a pizzeria – habits that often punctuate a night on the town. Don't use alcohol as a "vacation

from stress." That's like putting a Band-Aid on a gunshot wound. Find healthy, sustainable ways to deal with stress. And one great way to burn off that stress is definitely exercise!

After speaking with this diet and exercise guru, it's more evidence that shows you're not stuck in a body that's unsatisfying. Brett literally had a metamorphosis that makes him unrecognizable from his childhood. I see this type of transformation happen with people all the time, but it starts with a clear goal, willingness to change, and commitment. Take stock of your habits and see if you're slipping up in any of these areas. Are you willing to modify your diet and exercise routine? Can you cut back on the drinking? How about making sleep a priority? If the answer is YES, don't feel bad about it. Embrace this information and let it motivate you. Just don't wait too long!

CHAPTER 15

OH THE JOY OF HORMONES

How annoying is it when you decide to start a diet with your boyfriend or significant other and after two weeks he has lost ten pounds and you've only lost two? Hormones may be to blame. I've worked with several medical practices that specialized in weight loss protocols. Yet the men almost always lost significantly more than the women following exactly the same program. Your first thought could be, well since men weigh more than women then they will automatically lose more. That's not necessarily the case. Here are some reasons why hormones could be holding you back.

Estrogen Dominance Since women produce more estrogen, that keeps us storing fat in a different way than men do. Women who are estrogen dominant will have a hard time losing weight even when dieting. Some clues to determine if you may be estrogen dominant are PMS signs such as heavy periods, weight gain, mood swings, and loss of sex drive. With all the plastics and chemicals used in foods today, we are being given hefty doses of xenoestrogens from sources we may not even realize such as skin lotions, sunscreens, food colorings, insecticides, and microwaving food in plastic containers. Before you become symptomatic, the practice of checking your skin products for parabens, eating organic foods without chemicals and heating/storing your food in non-plastic containers is a little more work but definitely recommended.

Low Thyroid Function Thyroid disorders are especially prevalent in women and impact their ability to lose weight. The thyroid is like your internal thermostat and governs your metabolism. While some women have hyperthyroidism - which is an overactive thyroid - the most common thyroid disorder is hypothyroidism (under-active) thyroid or Hashimoto's Disease. Hashimoto's is when your body swings from hypothyroid to hyperthyroid. As someone who has experienced all the above thyroid conditions in addition to thyroid cancer, I urge you to check out your levels, especially if you can't lose weight.

Essentially, you can be doing all the cleansing and healthy eating you like, but if your thyroid is not doing its job you will not get very far. Not only can hypothyroidism cause you to be puffy, retain water and gain weight, it will make you so sluggish that you won't be motivated to exercise. Thyroid function is generally treated after assessing your TSH. TSH stands for Thyroid Stimulating Hormone. The acceptable range on a lab test is somewhere between 0.4-4.0 although physicians are finding that the more suppressed the TSH, the better the patient usually feels in terms of energy and metabolic rate. So you can have a blood test with a TSH level of 3.5 and find that although you have all the symptoms of hypothyroidism, you are still within the "normal" range. There are also some people don't feel well if their TSH is above a 2. You need to have a conversation with your doctor if your results fall into the upper quadrant of normal range and sense something is not right. The other tests to ask for are Free T4, Free T3 and Reverse T3 thyroid antibodies. While some endocrinologists discount these tests, unexplained weight gain and fatigue could be related to being out of balance.

Oral Contraception Birth control pills obviously have benefits, yet the drawbacks may not be worth it. In addition to loading your body with synthetic hormones, weight gain is a common side effect. Some women rely on the pill solely to prevent a pregnancy mishap; there are tons of women, however, who stay on it for Poly Cystic Ovary Syndrome (PCOS), acne or to ease PMS. While the pill won't make everyone gain weight, just know that the last 8-10 pounds that you can't lose can very likely be related. I've worked with young women that have been using the pill since their teenage years for their skin and swear by it. Yet they complain to me about not being the size they want. If that is the only reason they choose to use it, I try to see how they do being off the pill while making major dietary modifications. Many times they are eating too much sugar, yeast or processed foods. Once they clean up their diet, the skin will look better on its own. The weight comes off easier not being on the extra hormones and cutting out the unhealthy foods also helps to rev up the process.

You have to be your own detective to see if there is a root cause to failed dieting attempts. Tell your primary care physician that you want to complete a workup of your hormones. I generally ask to see lab work before working with someone to get the whole picture of what is going on. If a client is a vegan and I now find that's she's hypothyroid, I already see that to be a red flag. Soy products further inhibit thyroid function and so do even the healthiest of vegetables coming from the cruciferous vegetable family (i.e., kale, Brussels Sprouts, cauliflower, broccoli). It's not that you shouldn't ever eat these vegetables again, but they should be eaten in normal quantities. Juicing these vegetables on a regular basis can overburden the system rather than having a kale salad or some steamed broccoli once or twice a week.

Elizabeth, an interior decorator in her early thirties came to me complaining of low energy, lack of concentration and being unable to lose weight despite her "healthy vegetarian diet" and daily green juices. Since she was self-employed and didn't have health insurance, she assumed that her style of eating was the best preventative measure for not getting sick down the road.

During our first visit, Elizabeth confidently ran through her food choices. The only thing that she knew wasn't perfect was her 3-4 cups of coffee daily with soymilk to keep her going. Breakfast was usually cereal with almond or soy milk. Lunch was a salad with little protein except for maybe some chickpeas and a coffee. Later she would have a mid-afternoon kale juice. Dinner would be the biggest meal. It could be some kind of bean burrito on a whole grain wrap or soy product with vegetables and a large serving of rice or quinoa. Her vegetables of choice were always kale, broccoli and spinach.

Elizabeth had all the symptoms of hypothyroidism or possibly estrogen dominance, yet it couldn't be confirmed since she didn't want to pay out of pocket for her lab work. Being tired, bloated and unable to exercise shouldn't have been present for someone who was eating health foods all day long. The first thing I asked her to do was get off the coffee. I was concerned with the excessive caffeine raising her cortisol and insulin levels. Combined with her high carbohydrate diet and not enough protein, she was setting herself up for a metabolic disaster.

With some hesitation, she was willing to substitute her coffee for green tea. This actually worked since the small amount of caffeine from the tea gave her enough energy and allowed her to wean without headaches. Rather than a wheat and soy filled breakfast, I switched her over to organic eggs with vegetables or Greek yogurt with berries. On the go, she would make a protein shake (with low sugar fruit) in just eight ounces of water or mixed with unsweetened almond milk.

She got used to having a mid-morning snack to stabilize her blood sugar and keep her alert rather than grab another coffee. Usually it was a few raw almonds and an herbal tea which led her to not be starving at lunch time.

For lunch Elizabeth was again encouraged to have more protein than she was currently eating. She continued with salads and vegetables but we added fish, eggs, or feta cheese so she would be satisfied and not reach for another snack within an hour after her meal. Since Elizabeth was used to a high carbohydrate diet, it was a very big shift to make her eliminate most grains and starches. Small amounts of quinoa, sweet potato or brown rice were still recommended – but during the day rather than the evening for better weight loss results.

She still juiced, but I told her not to include the cruciferous vegetables such as kale and cabbage. Cucumber, celery, parsley, ginger and lemon were the ingredients best for her and also helped with digestion and water retention.

To keep full without the normal carb-laden dinners, Elizabeth added more healthy fats to her meals instead. I asked her to start with a salad and cook her vegetables in high quality olive oil along with a protein that would satisfy her. She didn't want to give up the soy protein completely, but I had her limit the tofu and tempeh to two days a week. She was also open to fish or even an omelet at night with her vegetables.

Within three months Elizabeth had lost ten pounds and with much more energy. Her cravings for sugar and coffee had almost completely disappeared and she didn't look as bloated. Yet she had reached a plateau. She finally got her insurance and had a complete lab work up which showed that she was slightly hypothyroid. With the help of a good endocrinologist, she started with a little thyroid hormone and within another month she had lost another seven pounds.

Don't just rely on a Google search to self-diagnose or follow the latest diet trend. What has worked for your friends may be completely counterproductive for your success. If you were trying to get pregnant and you had one failed attempt after the next, wouldn't you visit the doctor and find out if you were fertile or even ovulating? It would be silly to keep on having sex hoping for a different result before ruling out any underlying cause. The same applies to losing weight.

You can follow the most restrictive of diets, yet if your metabolism is compromised due to a hormonal issue, you could be totally wasting your time with so much unnecessary suffering. On the flip side, take responsibility for your lifestyle and don't blame a lazy thyroid for your size. You need to have confirmation either way. Go back to square one, have your hormones tested, and find out what's going on.

CHAPTER 16

UNCOVERING FOOD SENSITIVITIES

I used to say that the day I felt the best the entire year was on the holiday of Yom Kippur. Yes, I get hungry from a 24-hour fasting period but my stomach never bothers me, I sleep extremely well (which is rare), and I'm the clearest mentally. For the longest time - even when I felt like I was extremely cautious and health conscious with my diet - after meals in general I wouldn't feel great. If I knew that I had an important meeting, had to give a lecture, or perform in some sense, I would wait until after that engagement was over before eating or drinking anything other than water. I never wanted to risk feeling bloated, cramping, tired, spaced out or even anxious.

If specific foods are meant to nourish us, then why did I always have some sort of weird reaction after eating? I'm sure you know what I'm talking about. It's like when you eat something super healthy such as broccoli or Brussels sprouts and then blame your dog for the gas cloud in your apartment. I realized I was suffering from food sensitivities and they happen to be quite common. Different than true food allergies, food sensitivities are annoying but fortunately not life-threatening. The issue is that food sensitivities are hard to pinpoint since they often show up many hours after eating or drinking something that you're sensitive to. You could have a breakfast that's problematic which may not even affect you until late in the day or in the evening. Symptoms such as (IBS) irritable bowel syndrome, headaches, skin problems, fatigue, insomnia, etc. can come on mysteriously yet you most likely won't need an Epi-Pen or have to run to the emergency room.

Remember those little pin pricks going into your back as a kid to test for allergies? Well I do and believe me I was terrified of the doctor. What I had done was called the (RAST) Radioallergosorbent Test and it measured what are called (IgE) Immunoglobulin E antibodies. These antibodies are associated with true food allergies. Then there are other blood tests that look for food sensitivities which are detected by different antibodies called (IgG) Immunoglobulin G antibodies. Two blood tests that we commonly use in our office to check for food sensitivities are the ALCAT Test and The Pinner Test. When we have food sensitivities, they cause antibodies to be deposited into our tissues. The body tries to fight them off by causing inflammation which may be the root of our unpleasant symptoms. And remember, too much inflammation and weight gain go hand in hand.

Many foods that are healthy can still be problematic if you can't digest them. Some people lack the enzymes to break down specific foods. In this case the intolerance to those foods may be more permanent. For instance, if your body does not produce enough of the enzyme called lactase to break down lactose found in dairy products, this is a perfect example of how an intolerance begins. Just having one cup of milk can cause stomach bloating, gurgling, cramps and diarrhea. While lactose Intolerance is a worldwide phenomenon, there are many other intolerances that are not as obvious. We also know that in recent years there has been a movement against wheat and gluten due to their allergenic effects. Other foods commonly linked to allergies or intolerance are:

- Peanuts
- Tree nuts (almonds, walnuts, pistachios, pecans, cashews)
- Soy

- Eggs
- Yeast (found in most commercial breads, soups, dressings, sauces and baked goods)
- Citrus fruits (oranges, lemon, lime, grapefruit)
- Shellfish
- Night shade vegetables (potato, tomato, eggplant and peppers)

Sorry if that sounds pretty depressing and those foods make up the bulk of your diet. It doesn't mean you have to stop eating all those things if they are your world. And it's not always just narrowed down to the usual suspects. We need to also be aware of these factors in addition to the actual foods themselves:

- Preservatives
- Overload of naturally occurring chemicals in foods such as the caffeine in coffee, tea or chocolate, Xenoestrogens excreted from plastics
- Chemicals, chlorine, fluoride, heavy metals and antibiotics in our water
- Glyphosate (a toxin) which is sprayed on our fruits and vegetables
- Genetically modified versions of our foods

Now that it seems the environment for our food supply is totally screwed, there is still a way to detoxify from being overburdened from every direction. By making some modifications, not only will we feel better, but weight loss may follow. Food allergies and sensitivities are recognized by the body as toxins. The more chemicals and toxins your body is holding on to, this will cause fluid retention, swelling, and toxic build-up storing in your fat cells. Continual exposure to foods that your body can't tolerate eventually beats up your immune system, making it harder to stay healthy, in shape and feel good if you never give your body a break. With multiple food sensitivities, you become more susceptible to having frequent colds, yeast infections, and chronic headaches since you're constantly being bombarded.

As mentioned earlier, there are lab tests to detect food sensitivities. Yet they are not always 100% accurate. When you have an IgG food sensitivity - unlike an IgE food allergy - it's possible your results can change depending on when you take the test. Results can vary through the course of several months. I've seen many cases where a client's report shows multiple sensitivities and after following three months of avoiding those foods totally, they come up clear of those sensitivities on the next lab test. True food allergies are usually something you have for a lifetime, whereas sensitivities can come and go. Some women even have temporary food intolerances from hormonal changes that come on mysteriously before their period, mid-cycle or during or after pregnancy.

While lab testing can be a useful indicator for what foods may be bothering you or contributing to weight gain, there is a less clinical way of figuring it out on your own. Many physicians I've worked with have created their own versions of what we call an "Elimination Diet." I've worked with some of the New York based leaders in the field of detoxification including Dr. Jeffrey Morrison and Oz Garcia. (I have had the latter's mentoring for several years and currently see clients at his office.) Additionally – and although he has never been a colleague - I think Dr. Alejandro Junger has a terrific detoxification protocol called the "Clean Program." All three of these programs are what I consider to be the Gold Standard of safe cleansing and clearing symptoms of food sensitivities.

The protocol involves drinking a Detox shake 1-3 times a day in the place of a meal. There are a few brands we've worked with, but typically the shake would be high in protein while carrying low-allergenic potential. Usually it would also be based from rice. These formulations contain amino acids that support detoxification and antioxidants which prevent typical detox side effects that may be experienced from, say, just drinking a green juice or lemon water during a fast. Professional lines that are primarily sold to physicians have the most trusted shakes. Any of these companies make a superior shake to a store-bought brand during a food sensitivity elimination diet.

- Thorne Research - MediClear Plus®
- Metagenics - UltraClear® Plus
- Xymogen® - OptiCleanse™

The goal is to eliminate potentially toxic foods or those foods you consider to be suspect from your diet for a period of weeks. Included in this not so fun (but well worth it) experience are the following foods:

- Processed foods: Anything in a box, bag, can, or frozen (with the exclusion of plain frozen fruits and vegetables)
- Nightshade vegetables: Potato, tomato, eggplant and peppers (since they are inflammatory)
- Sugar and artificial sweeteners: Stevia™ is okay
- Dairy products (milk, cheese, whey, yogurt, cottage cheese)
- Wheat and gluten: Stay away from gluten-free versions if trying to lose weight (i.e., bread, pasta or pastries made from rice or potato flour)
- Soy (tofu, tempeh, soybeans, edamame)
- Coffee: It creates inflammation which contributes to weight gain. (switch over to green tea)
- Alcohol (wine, beer and mixed drinks are loaded with sugar and yeast)

For the best success, stay as organic as possible. Although expensive, organic selections will free you up from worrying about GMO's, pesticides, hormones and antibiotics creeping into our food. Make sure to drink lots of clean, purified water – never from the tap and free of flavorings or carbonation. Once you start adding artificial sweeteners to water or bubbles, it becomes acidic. Fresh water helps to alkalize and detoxify the system while excreting all the by-products from things that are irritating us.

How the allergy elimination diet works:
Breakfast Mix one of the non-allergenic Detox powders I listed with purified water. You can add ½ cup berries as long as they are organic.

Lunch Have another shake and you can add large servings of organic vegetables with the exception of "Nightshade Vegetables" (remember they can cause inflammation). Additionally, no corn or peas since they are very starchy and will not help if you are trying to lose weight. Don't be afraid to use healthy oils such as olive oil or flaxseed oil. They will actually lubricate the system and aid in the elimination process.

Dinner This is the meal that you don't have to use the shake. Organic chicken, turkey, or wild-caught fish should be your main protein. Just watch eating tuna more than once per week due to the high mercury content. Shrimp, lobster, crab and shellfish may contain sulfites and should be avoided. In fact, any shellfish is general could be a problem so leave it alone for the time being. Lean cuts of lamb or beef are okay once per week (preferably grass-fed and organic). Vegetarians can eat beans or lentils that have been soaked overnight. Pour out the water and rinse before cooking.

Every meal including dinner should have sufficient amounts of organic vegetables either drizzled in oil or steamed. The same rules apply to when you eat them at lunchtime.

What about starches and grains with meals?

Non-gluten containing grains such as quinoa, brown rice, wild rice, or amaranth can go with any meal. Butternut squash makes a great side too. Yet if you are doing this program to lose weight in addition to eliminate food sensitivities, make sure to eat grains or any starch in modest amounts and early in the day.

When to reintroduce foods back into the diet:

The first few days of eliminating most of the foods you are addicted to it will most likely be rough. It's normal to have cravings, feel a little tired, perhaps even experience a pubescent break out. That all can be part of the detoxification process. After a week, most people feel more energized, have better digestion, their skin clears up, headaches come on less frequently and they just look better. The body gets a break from being inflamed and, as a result, weight loss usually occurs.

Since it's not realistic to stay on a restricted program for a prolonged period of time, you will eventually start reintroducing foods back in the diet. The best way to do this is to start a journal. Do each food one by one. Don't just go back to your old ways and add everything back all at once since you won't know what is making you sensitive if you have a reaction. For the first week you may reintroduce eggs. If you feel okay with them, week two you may decide to bring back yogurt. Then week three you may want to have some tomatoes (which are part of the nightshade family) with your eggs. If at that point you feel sensitive, you can then determine that the tomatoes are bothering you and not the eggs so much. Keep doing this slowly and work to be in tune with your body.

For long-term prevention:

As a lifestyle, it's best to add variety to your meals. If you are susceptible to food intolerance and eat the same foods every day, it's likely you will develop a sensitivity to them – even if they are healthy. The way to prevent reactions is by rotating your foods. If you like oatmeal for breakfast, then have it two days in a row a week and then no oatmeal again for the next four days. The same rotation method goes for eating chicken at lunch or salmon at dinner. Having these "off" days in-between can help you tolerate foods that were once troublesome. Yet if you continue to eat them daily, your issues may arise again.

Get creative with your meal planning and even seek out a nutritionist if you need some guidance along the way. It takes some preparation and planning ahead, but with the right maintenance you can continue to feel good and keep the weight off.

CHAPTER 17

BIG BELLY - BAD BACTERIA

There is a new spin on obesity that people are first beginning to understand. Before blaming weight gain on lack of self-control or laziness, recent research suggests that the bacteria in our gut may be a key contributor. Mike Mutzel, holds a Master of Science degree in nutrition and is the author of *Belly Fat Effect*. Since this is such a hot topic, I wanted to get his feedback on what we can do to improve our intestinal bacteria to help us burn fat. (Mike's comments are below in italics.)

Gut health has been a central part of traditional Asian medicine for centuries, yet it's something that we've almost completely ignored in Western science. The trillions of microbes in our gut can be associated with chronic inflammation which often leads to autoimmune disease, insulin resistance, diabetes, depression, allergies, heart disease, and weight gain. The importance of the quality of our intestinal flora is often something we never think about. Every day through the foods we eat, the alcohol we love, and the medications or antibiotics we rely on but perhaps don't need, we have the ability to improve our gut bacteria or destroy it.

Studies reveal that obese people tend to have lower levels of bacterial diversity (especially the good kind). Instead they have greater levels of intestinal bacteria overgrowth and often unhealthy intestinal methane-producing bacteria. This can slow down food transit time and prolong the time intestinal bacteria are exposed to food. As a result, more calories are absorbed from that food and what do you think happens? Yes, it's weight gain. This can explain why just eating fewer calories may not always be the solution to weight loss if there are imbalances in your gut.

Where does a healthy gut begin?

Researchers have discovered that babies born vaginally and also breast fed have an advantage in the development of healthy gut microflora. During the birthing process, the babies become inoculated with the mother's vaginal flora - which is extremely healthy for the baby. Breast milk is also rich in beneficial bacteria that get transmitted to the infant. It's no mistake that our body is designed in this way to give the best possible chance of health and survival to our offspring. There has been so much to support this theory that in 2011 the Centers for Disease Control and Prevention (CDC) endorsed breast feeding as a prevention against obesity, suggesting that nursing could decrease the odds by 30 percent that the child would become obese.

We can also put ourselves at a disadvantage when we have low levels of an enzyme called alkaline phosphatase. Harvard scientists found that alkaline phosphatase may be a critical component of keeping gut microbes in check. When a person continually eats a processed, high-fat diet, this enzyme can be depleted. Additionally, alkaline phosphatase functions better in a more alkaline environment instead of one that is acidic. Fruits and green leafy vegetables tend to keep the body alkaline, yet we shift to a more acidic body when eating lots of meat, using artificial sweeteners, refined carbohydrates, hard cheeses and too many medications. Alkaline phosphatase can help us preserve healthy microbes while stunting the growth of some of the more problematic ones. When these bad bacteria are prevalent, they can alter the strength of the intestinal wall and lead to leaky gut syndrome. Leaky gut activates a variety of immune messengers, which alter insulin. Insulin is a critical hormone involved in metabolism and the way the body uses digested food for energy. Leaky gut can lead to insulin resistance - causing glucose to build up in the blood instead of being absorbed by the cells. Down the road that can end up leading to type 2 diabetes or prediabetes.

Since we don't have control over the way our mothers delivered or fed us as babies, Mike is clear about the importance of what we can manage – especially food quality and the role it plays in our gut ecosystem. Even if a fast food or chain restaurant offers a diet menu – such as low-fat or low-carb offerings - this does not qualify those meals as being healthy. Turkey sausage or bacon, chicken breast, or egg whites to swap out their more fattening alternatives can still be hazardous to our health if they have been pumped up with antibiotics. If you are constantly consuming animal products that are not organic, the antibiotics administered can be passed through the meat and could potentially change your microbiome. Without diversity in the foods you eat, there becomes less diversity in your gut bacteria.

Let's say you wanted to follow a very low-carbohydrate diet - eating three bacon cheeseburgers per day without a bun and a couple diet sodas. There are people who actually do this to lose weight and think they are not doing damage because they are technically not going over their allotted limit of calories or carbohydrates. To make matters worse, they then go home and top it off with chemically engineered desserts such as fat-free frozen yogurt, sugar-free pudding or Jell-O™. Besides all the saturated fat, cholesterol, and artificial sweeteners, this bombardment of toxicity would be making a mess of your gut ecology.

A study performed in 2015 by The British Gut Project and Cornell University showed how eating just 10 days straight of McDonald's can change your gut bacteria. The son of a college professor went on a diet of Big Macs™, Chicken nuggets, fries and Coke™. He sent his stool samples to different labs and when he got his results back, findings showed that he had lost about 40 percent of his gut bacteria species. So if this happened in just a little over a week, can you imagine what years of eating this way can do?

How can we restore our gut bacteria to prevent future weight gain?

As mentioned before with the fast food example, anything that our bodies perceive as toxic can destroy gut flora and damage our intestines. We know that high-fat foods and processed meats can be problematic, but how about grains? Most modern day foods like cookies, pastries, bagels, pretzels, cereal, and any other refined grains are especially responsible for destroying our gut bacteria. Wheat and gluten typically found in these foods both contain proteins that can damage the lining of the gut. Not to mention these foods are often baked with sugar, high fructose corn syrup and unhealthy oils.

The bottom line is that if what you're eating is not real food, there will be consequences. Numerous studies have demonstrated why the microbiome of people living in isolated societies is superior. The BBC News reported on the benefits of an African style diet (high-fiber and low-fat) as opposed to a Western Diet. Another story was published on the diversity in the microbiome of Amazonian Tribes in the Journal of Nature Communications. Additionally NPR News released a report on indigenous people and how their gut bacteria is close to the bacteria of our ancestors. None of these cultures have been exposed to the industrialization and tampering of foods that we have along with medications, antibiotics, etc.

Understand that sticking to natural ingredients rather than swapping out with artificial substitutes to save on calories will only slow us down in the long run. If our foundation (our gut) is not healthy, we are not being holistic about making a long lasting impact to our health and weight. As Mike Mutzel says, "Our intestinal flora is as impressionable as a child on a schoolyard playground. And food can change that playground." A fad diet can work temporarily, yet once the foundation is shaken - since we didn't nurture it in the first place - we'll keep bouncing from diet to diet for the rest of our lives. To face this issue head-on, we want to eat a diverse selection of organic foods in addition to many fruits and vegetables to keep our bacteria diverse.

We should also include in that variety foods that naturally contain prebitocs and probiotics to help our bacteria flourish. Prebiotics get the party started to make the probiotics work even better. Bananas, asparagus, onions and garlic are some basics that are easy to incorporate. For naturally occurring probiotics – plain yogurt, sauerkraut, pickled vegetables and if you are adventurous even kimchi is great. Lastly, nutritional supplements can be powerful players for added support. Mike recommends prebiotic and probitic supplements in addition to herbal compounds such as berberine, garlic, oregano and peppermint oil which can all work to repair gut health. Just make sure to check in with a healthcare professional before undergoing any new supplement regimen since you need to know the proper amounts to take before you overdo it. It's not like the more ammo you use, the more effective you will be at killing the bad guys.

In life it seems that everything comes down to the gut. That's why the gut is also known as "the second brain." You know when you have that "gut feeling" – good or bad - about something. Our brain and gut are in constant communication. Seventy to eighty percent of our immune system also lives there, determining the fate of our health. Once we understand how much of our emotional and physical health are ruled by the state of our gut, correcting this without question should be our first line of defense!

CHAPTER 18

THE PLIGHT OF THE ORTHOREXIC

As if there weren't already enough eating disorders out there, there is a now another condition that is spreading rampantly. It's called Orthorexia and the definition is a person who suffers from an unhealthy obsession with healthy eating. The condition came to be in 1997 by the author of *Health Food Junkies*, Dr. Steven Bratman. While Orthorexia is not considered an actual clinical diagnosis, the term is becoming very popular since we all probably know someone who falls into this category. It's easy to become victim to Orthorexic tendencies since there's often a sense of elitism and accomplishment that accompanies being a health freak. It feels very much like a private club that only the fittest can be part of.

While that doesn't seem so terrible, these individuals never veer off. And if they do, it comes with the same kind of guilt and shame as an alcoholic who just had a relapse or unprotected sex with a total stranger. Orthorexics can become completely anxiety-ridden about the implications of what may happen as a result of their one poor food choice. A few bites of a meal with refined sugar, gluten, or non-organic ingredients could provoke a serious breakdown.

So how does being too healthy sabotage your body? It almost sounds conflicting to the advice dispensed throughout this book. The reason is because extremes in any direction are never good. Think of it this way: Imagine someone you know who was an alcoholic and has now been sober for some time while attending regular meetings of Alcoholics Anonymous. The ex-alcoholic will often look at people who drink socially as being irresponsible even if they have a handle on their behavior. But are they really being irresponsible or just challenging the new belief system that the former alcoholic now has? The social drinker can most likely get through life while enjoying alcohol with little consequence because it's a pleasure and not an obsession. The person who is sober, however, fights a daily battle to not think about liquor. It consumes them. To fight off their inclinations, they may become more religious, take up mindfulness practices, become abstinent and then stand in judgment of their friends because, after all, they took control of their life and their friends are simply carefree and ignorant. This addictive behavior mirrors the mentality of the Orthorexic.

For them, "Superfoods" and "healthy habits" have taken the place of drinking. It's not uncommon to even see a former alcoholic become an Orthorexic since it's swapping one destructive behavior for another (disguised as something positive). Much of this condition is about control, discipline and achieving physical excellence. It's actually quite similar to anorexia except fat is not the enemy. Instead, it's sugar, anything processed and chemicals that assume the role of the devil. Orthorexics often stick to their guns about healthy eating habits as a weight loss method but it doesn't always work. Adding organic coconut oil to your coffee, making smoothies with hemp and cashew butter, snacking on chia seeds from an Amazonian tribe or special berries from Peru will not make you skinny.

Now let's clarify that there's a difference between being particular about the way you eat and being Orthorexic. I may come across as I'm promoting Orthorexia because many of my suggestions require giving up on certain indulgences and living a health conscious lifestyle. In the same regard, keeping your fridge stocked with low-fat and fat-free foods doesn't mean you are anorexic. My concern is that you work smart and not hard when it comes to losing weight. If you are going to put everything you eat under a microscope, at least make sure the pay-off is worth it. The worst examples I see of seemingly "diet" meals are on Pinterest or YouTube. Women often post recipes that are Orthorexic approved because they contain no artificial ingredients. Often stay at home moms (or people who have struggled with their own weight) will spend hours in the kitchen like chemists conjuring up meals that would otherwise contain processed ingredients with their picks for more natural food swaps. Social media is the place that they share all their discoveries, but don't run to copy those recipes so fast. Instead of making pancakes with regular flour, they'll create a buckwheat version. How about a burger made from beans and walnuts instead of red meat? Or as a substitute for ice cream you can now make a non-dairy milkshake of raw cashews, organic dates, manuka honey and unsweetened cocoa powder. Many are calorie bombs and most of these recipes that appear too good to be true usually are. Getting too creative in the food department can cause problems; sometimes it's better to keep it clean and simple.

Although I consult on nutrition for a living, if your life and social interests always revolve around food (even the healthy kind), it will end up backfiring. Now if you're one of those individuals that has been told you have food allergies, gluten intolerance, celiac, candida, etc. then yes you should be cautious (especially if there is a serious health consequence to a slip up). If you choose restriction as a preference, be careful not to become a hypochondriac because that has consequences also. Deciding to go strict Paleo, Vegan, Gluten-Free, Fruitarian, or Raw Foodist and never flexible in any circumstance can pose a risk. What the Orthorexic often fails to realize is that having perfect health and a killer body is not only a matter of pristine diet and exercise.

I can say this with certainty because I was somewhat of an Orthorexic in my past. I spoke a bit about this in my book *Smile At Your Challenges (It takes more than just going gluten free, drinking green juice and practicing yoga to solve your problems)*. When I was writing the book, I had never even heard the term Othorexic and thought I was alone in my need to be a perfect physical specimen free of any potential risk for illness. Since my mother died at 38 years old of breast cancer, I was committed to doing everything possible to not be like her and share the same fate.

In the early stages of my wellness career, I was one of those rah rah people that only ate things that were green or fell from a tree, and often did two workouts in one day. You know, like your friends that post photos every two hours on Instagram with messages like "Day 3 of my liver cleanse," "Just had the best colonic," or "Yoga rocked and I feel so one with myself!" I was no different except the app didn't exist yet to share social posts about my healthy activities.

Although I wasn't specifically focusing on my weight, I believed this was the path to self-improvement. Yet, truthfully I was no happier than I was before I went down that road. If anything, it made me very stressed around mealtimes and I came off as uptight. People would always feel the need to apologize for their eating habits in front of me. It took years to find my happy medium, yet I often see people go from being super rigid to letting go and falling off the wagon. This is a major issue for people who have had trouble with dieting in the first place. When they become overwhelmed with restriction, they can crack.

When clients work with me on their diet, I always allow them one cheat day. You can tell someone they can't have a bite of anything sweet for a month, but what happens when there is a sense of not being fulfilled and nothing to look forward to? Maybe you guessed it? Rebellion! If you are on a quest to lose weight and become Orthorexic in the process, you've just set yourself up for a heavy burden. If the reward was so great, or it was a guarantee you'd never get heart disease, cancer or anything troublesome, then perhaps there would be more gratification. Unfortunately, the consequences of an unhappy spirit will kill you faster than a little gluten or white sugar.

Before I ever became a full blown Orthorexic, I began developing severe health problems and got stopped in my tracks. Despite being extremely calculated with my healthy lifestyle, it was God, karma or the universe that was calling the shots. My issues began with vicious insomnia for weeks that no natural remedy could conquer. Chamomile tea, magnesium, and herbal remedies were child's play. Meditation was somewhat relaxing but after nights on end with no sleep, even that became irritating because I couldn't concentrate. The only thing that would knock me out required a prescription. Here I was - the poster child for clean living and I'm drugging myself to sleep every night. Once the insomnia finally became somewhat managed, the digestive problems kicked in. How does someone who doesn't eat wheat, inflammatory foods, dairy or anything processed feel like she has colitis? When I finally got to the root of my symptoms it turned out I had thyroid cancer. It was ironic - I dedicated my life to controlling every move to be healthy and yet was worse off than all of my friends.

In times of crisis, it makes you reflect on your life, how did you get there and what steps would you take to never repeat the same mistake. Before having my thyroid removed, I had never had any surgery or undergone anesthesia in my life. I rarely went to a doctor other than to just have a simple blood test.

My whole world was upside down from living 100% holistic to now taking medication daily and going under the knife. At one point I literally thought there was a chance I could die. I knew if there was hope for me to get through this, I'd chill out regarding my rigid eating and exercise habits going forward. I re-learned how to enjoy a glass of wine with friends, a piece of red meat because I have a craving, or some chocolate chip cookies when my period's coming on without feeling guilty. So long to the days of waking up at 5 a.m. in the winter to make it downtown to yoga on time. My 6 a.m. daily yoga practice turned into a self-practice at home when my body is in the mood without setting an alarm. On the other days I'll either go to the gym or take a long, leisurely walk based on how I feel that day. There's no feeling of "No pain no gain" rather just go with the flow. Like you, I'm a woman who cares about being thin, healthy and attractive. I have no shame in being pickier than others with my eating habits or exercising regularly, yet I came to the conclusion that it's okay to be bending and not make diet and fitness a religion. You don't have to put pressure on yourself to always be a Saint. Skewing your habits in a healthy direction lets you be sinful at times while still feeling good about it.

CHAPTER 19

HOW TO PARTY WITHOUT PAYING FOR IT

Although I may prefer to spend most Saturday nights these days over a quiet dinner rather than be out with cool plans, I still get the itch to let my hair down. The first club I ever went to was called the Limelight and it was the place to be in NYC during the 90's. No ID really required; it was more about being cool enough to get past the velvet rope. At just 14 years old I dressed in the most impressive outfit I owned. Being that I was a huge Madonna fan, I wore a long sleeved pinstriped half-top with, yes, "cone boobs." (Try to visualize her Blonde Ambition Tour.) To make this outfit more of a nightmare to anyone's parents, it was paired with short, patent leather boy shorts and six-inch platform shoes. My hair, of course, matched her signature high pony tail. I was a six-foot tall child trying to pass myself off as 21 as I confidently cut the line, walked to the front of it and was granted access by the doorman.

This process was so easy that clubbing became a thrill and regular pastime. Being that I was underage didn't prevent me from drinking alcohol. In fact, it was actually quite easy to access if someone else was buying. Initially, I really hadn't developed a taste for it unless it was something super sweet like a Cosmopolitan, Chocolate Martini or Long Island Iced Tea that masked the flavor. As the years went by and I grew into my late teens and early twenties, my palate became more sophisticated and I started to enjoy drinking. Going out also didn't start until really late. We rarely went to a club before 11 p.m. or midnight which meant we were pre- gaming at someone's apartment beforehand. Usually beers, vodka with juice, or wine were readily available. Maybe we'd even order a pizza while we were hanging out and have chips, pretzels and snack foods lying around. After a while I noticed the puffy face and a bloated belly.

It's one thing to be on good behavior in your own company, yet it's hard to step up to peer pressure when everyone else is being indulgent. You don't have to be in a sorority to get yourself into this kind of trouble. Trust me; the invitations for debauchery are still flowing every night even now in my 30's. Regardless if you plan to stay out until 4 in the morning dancing all night, you won't burn off enough calories to undo the damage. Another fun fact: even if you get lucky over the course of the night, a study by the University of Montreal reveals that the average calories a woman expends during sex is just 69! (Weird number I know.) That may be about only a half a drink.

You could have a personal trainer that challenges you every single day and maybe keep up a fairly decent diet, yet if you have a free-for-all more than one night a week it's going to be really difficult to see any progress. How you end your nights is as important as how you start your days. I have a couple of party ground rules I never break. It's like a personal oath that has allowed me to have fun for the past 20 years without letting my body suffer for it. Not only will maintaining these habits keep you from gaining weight but will also keep you from looking worn out and tired.

1. **Never leave home feeling hungry** If your plan is to have cocktails at a friend's house before your night out, make sure you have eaten something substantial. A meal high in protein is the best

since it will keep your blood sugar balanced and not tempted to snack later. Don't go out somewhere expecting that they will be serving food so you don't need to eat in advance. They most likely will be serving food but nothing your body will be happy about. If you had a good dinner, you shouldn't feel hungry. Hors d'oeuvres are off limits other than vegetable crudités. This means cheese, pretzels, popcorn, dumplings, chicken fingers, etc. These foods will put you in the danger zone. In your mind, pretend you are allergic and do not touch. Once you take your first bite, it's hard to stop and your diet has been blown.

2. **Keep it clean and clear** Wine, beer, champagne, juice, tonic and any kind of premade drink mix is a trap. Learn to acquire a taste for vodka or tequila on the rocks, neat, with water, club soda or muddled with fresh lemons and limes. Just know that these drinks are strong and drinking like a man may get you a little messy. Make sure to pace yourself and nurse each beverage. Don't chug it down like "Girls gone wild" or you won't make it to the next party. Walk around a little just to make sure you're not stumbling or saying anything that doesn't make sense. In between each drink, have a glass of water to stay hydrated. If you have a long night ahead of you, please don't have more than one drink per destination. And ideally you shouldn't have more than two drinks a night (not every night either). Not only should you be concerned about alcohol calories, but also the toxicity associated with making drinking a habit and a crutch to be able to enjoy going out. If you want to space it out, have half a drink at each location. If you find that partying is boring without drinking, then congratulations! That means you're probably maturing and should find more productive ways to spend your free time.

3. **Do not smoke pot** I hope you choose to never mess around with drugs. Yet since marijuana is becoming legal in so many states and viewed less harmless than say cocaine, Molly (Ecstasy), or any kind of stimulant, it has become a big party favorite. While pot can help you let go of inhabitations and make the dumbest comment sound like the most hysterical thing you've ever heard, it's all fun and games until your brain starts to go, you lose judgment and can't pull your shit together. Then once the munchies kick in for brownies, chocolate chip cookies, or some treat that a nine year old would buy with their allowance, there's no turning back!
4. **Make your exit by 1 a.m.** Honestly, nothing good usually happens past midnight. If you are out for networking purposes, all the important movers and shakers have already left because they have work or responsibilities the following morning or a family to go home to. Any guy who is hitting you up at the wee hours of the night is probably already hammered and does not want to go home alone. You don't want to be the low-hanging fruit. More important than staying out until dawn is to get your beauty sleep and potentially a worthwhile workout the following morning.
5. **Keep strict bedtime rituals** If you keep to the program and don't snack during the course of the night, chances are you will feel like you need something in your system. That's fine; just don't eat anything high in carbohydrates before bed. Politely decline the invitations for late night pizza or hot and toasty bagels with friends and don't do the lazy bowl of cereal thing when you get home. Plan ahead and make sure to have hardboiled eggs, turkey slices, chicken breast or Greek yogurt in your fridge to the rescue. Additionally, it may be a good idea to take a magnesium supplement before retiring. Magnesium helps to relax the body which

is beneficial after partying while feeling so awake and stimulated. Magnesium also helps relieve constipation which will push out the toxins. Combining magnesium and a powerful probiotic supplement will decrease inflammation caused from drinking and restore healthy bacteria to your digestive system.

There's no reason why you can't party and have fun if you feel like it. If you've worked so hard on getting into shape, then you deserve to dress up and show yourself off. Just make sure you plan ahead and you're conscious throughout the course of the night. It may seem a little much to always have to be on guard, but with healthy moderation you can keep the party going for the next 50 years!

CHAPTER 20

THE RIGHT TRACK TO SUCCESS

We live in the informational age. With the press of a button, it has become incredibly simple to learn about anything you put into your body and break down its nutrients on a microscopic level. This is the generation of electronics and gadgets to help you track every physical aspect of your day which can be especially beneficial when keeping tabs on your weight. After my first session with clients, I give them a bit of homework; specifically, to track their progress. The cool part is that everything can be shared with me electronically and reviewed together in subsequent meetings.

Whether you use your smart phone, a wrist band, or a watch that looks as if you double as a secret agent, these devices can keep tabs on the nutritional profile of the foods you eat, amount of exercise you're getting, calories burned after activities or even the number of hours that you sleep.

I remember when I was a nutraceutical rep and used to call on doctors as my accounts. In the beginning, my boss would ask how many prospects I saw in a day. I would usually come up with some ballpark figure and tell him everything looked promising. Then came the time that if I hadn't come through with as any deals as expected or didn't hit my goals, he started requesting a spreadsheet. It made me panic because now I had to be accountable. It's easy to say, "Oh yeah everything is great. I'm doing all I can on my part and visit tons of doctors' offices but I can't figure out why I'm not hitting my targets." The truth was, a part of me was lazy. It's not like I didn't believe in my products, didn't want to be more successful or make big commissions. I definitely needed the extra money. But I knew that if I put forth at least some effort (even if it wasn't focused) maybe I'd get lucky. It's like throwing spaghetti against the wall and hoping it sticks.

The first day I was required to start logging, it was a bit scary. I know I presented to him that I saw a minimum of 5-6 doctors daily, but were they true appointments or was I just dropping off samples to the front desk girl at random offices and guessing/hoping/assuming those samples would get into the right hands? Not only did I now have to say who I met with but also jot notes on what was discussed and the anticipated timelines for follow-up and sales. As I reviewed my interactions, it made me realize I was lying to myself. I was always complaining about how I have so many bills, how expensive it is to live in NY and why it wasn't fair I was spending my entire day running all over town and still not getting paid my worth for the amount of time I committed to this job. Yet I wasn't doing the actual work to change my circumstance. Had I taken more direction and made a focused effort, I could have been making an uncapped amount of money. Only when the full case was presented in my face did I actually see where I was failing and, as a result, my new awareness shifted my efforts and led to a huge growth in new accounts.

This is typically the scenario when I'm working with a client and we're not seeing progress. They might say something like, "I only eat a small breakfast, just some salad for lunch and then fish and vegetables for dinner. It's not like I have a sweet tooth, either. Then I go to the gym almost every day." Being that I don't have anyone under 24-hour surveillance, I have to take their word for it. It makes my job difficult because I'm not always sure what to say to that seemingly perfect effort. If someone is paying you, it's a little overstepping boundaries to interrogate them to uncover why the results don't add up – unlike your boss who has the right to question your lack of success.

My solution to cutting through the BS? It's all about tracking. Yes, it requires some homework but the picture becomes much clearer for both parties. I want to know what you are eating and drinking for breakfast, lunch and dinner, what you go for at snack time and if you slip up before bed. What kind of physical activity you are up to, how many hours are you sleeping and are you eliminating every day or plugged up and constipated. Asking for all this information can seem a bit intrusive. Without this full transparency, however, lying to yourself or any practitioner you work with will just delay major improvements.

I suggest several apps depending on the client's preference to share information. As we go through each day together, something like this typically happens with my commentary:

Breakfast Non-fat Greek yogurt and berries for breakfast. **Me** "*Ok that's good*" Caramel Macchiato **Me** "*I thought you said you have coffee every morning*" **Her** "*That is my coffee- I don't like the taste of plain coffee, it's too bitter*" Already I see this is adding on extra calories.

Snack Dried fruit and granola. **Me** "*I thought you don't really snack.* **Her** "*Well I don't snack on anything junky like potato chips or cookies but sometimes I keep a bag of granola and dried fruit at my desk because it's healthy and it's allows me to take a later lunch*" She doesn't realize that this particular snack can be as caloric as an actual lunch.

Lunch Salad with tuna, avocado, walnuts, chickpeas, feta cheese, dried cranberries, and olive oil dressing. **Me** "*Did you make this salad at home or was it from a café?*" **Her** "*From the café our office orders from all the time. It's a pretty light lunch and I never have bread.*" While all the ingredients in the salad are reasonably healthy, I have to dissect this kind of lunch. There are multiple proteins which should be spread out through different meals. Walnuts can be a snack on their own, the feta cheese can be a protein with dinner and I would limit the salad to just tuna and avocado with additional greens. Chickpeas have some protein but tend to be very starchy and unless you are serving yourself, the café can over serve you with 2-3 portions. Additionally, dried cranberries have tons of sugar and chances are these are not organic and have artificial ingredients and sulfites. To top it off, the amount of olive oil used to dress your salad can be tremendous. So now your harmless salad could be over 1000 calories while loaded with fat and sugar!

Snack Hummus and baby carrots. **ME** *"Okay, that's a good snack- how much did you eat?"* **Her** *"Maybe a half a bag of carrots and a small container of hummus from Whole Foods."* **Me** *"Right, carrots are nutritious and have many vitamins, but did you realize a serving of hummus is two tablespoons and a container is about seven servings?* That snack could be close to 700 calories.

Dinner Grilled salmon and vegetables with quinoa. **Me** *"I'm happy with that dinner."*

Snack Raw chocolate squares, grapes and then some cashews. *"Was that all at the same time?"* **Her** *"No, it's throughout the night. I like to go to sleep late and sometimes get the munchies but I don't eat anything bad."* My radar automatically goes off and I think did she eat a bar of chocolate, a bowl of grapes or a bag of cashews? What are we talking here? This can be another few hundred to over a thousand calories.

Exercise 30 minutes of walking and climbing stairs **Me** *"Was this brisk walking? What kind of stairs were you climbing?* **Her** *"I walk to and from the subway to work every day which is 15 minutes each direction - 30 minutes total and I live in a 5-floor walk up and don't use the elevator."* We get into a discussion how cardio needs to be consistent for a prolonged period of time to be effective. Not broken up into 15 minute intervals such as walking from Times Square to your office and back (only a few avenues each direction). Walking up five flights of stairs is a good habit, but is not necessarily going to burn off the pounds.

Sleep 6 Hours. **Me** *"Could you have gotten more sleep?"* **Her** *"Yes, was just up late watching TV and on the computer."* Going to sleep earlier could have prevented late night snacking.

Elimination Feeling like digestion is very slow. **Me** *"Are you drinking enough water?"* **Her** *"Water is a little too plain so I drink seltzer or flavored waters."* Clean water is essential to purify the body and eliminate toxins (i.e., relieving constipation). Seltzer, carbonated beverages and sports drinks don't have the same detoxifying benefits.

Look what's wrong with this situation. Do you think there's a part of you that can relate? Before you give up and assume with certainty that nothing will work, tracking has to be step #1. Once you've logged all of your daily information, trust me it will be more apparent where the problem lies. In this case, her caloric intake exceeded her estimation by more than double. These habits seemed so harmless that they would probably have been missed through conversations in the first few consults. What you thought qualified as exercise may have not made a dent and you may have also come to realize that you could sleep better, feel less stressed and less toxic. Most people are not in touch with their bodies so it's no surprise that half our population is overweight. Without these tracking devices, you can keep going in circles and not understanding why you are fated to a body that won't change. Please be certain that's not the case. What I want to stress is that you shouldn't be upset if you come to realize that you've been going about your weight loss attempts all wrong. This is actually the opposite and should be viewed as a blessing. I'm always thrilled when I work with clients and we figure out where mistakes were being made. This only means that we can make corrections and repair the damage.

Ladies, tomorrow is a new day. Let's break those "fat girl habits"!

Made in the USA
Middletown, DE
10 April 2017